My Dear Woman, You Aren't Crazy
The Change is Real
No More Shame
Knowledge is Power
Story, Sip, Science, Strategy
Fantastic Four
Definitions

Acknowledgments

To write, publish, and market a book is a daunting task—one full of self-doubt, challenges to overcome, extreme highs and lows, and learning repeatedly what you don't know you don't know. Then you shift and pivot and seemingly go backwards to move forward. The support of a few important people in my life helped me birth this book.

First, I thank my writing coach and book editor, Ben Allen. His encouragement and ability to key into what I needed at different points in the process was invaluable. He kept me writing, thinking, and editing and gave me hope that, yes, this would get finished, and it would be worthy to put out into the world.

Kristen Yates, heard my "voice" immediately and gave me editing suggestions and ideas to stay consistent with my message.

In the writing department, I also must thank my mentor Ann Sheybani (annsheybani.com). Her book, How to Eat the Elephant, was my guide. She breaks down how to write a book succinctly, and the step-by-step process helped me immensely.

My friend and restaurateur, Christopher Holland, owner of Taproot Lounge and Café, generously shared his mixology expertise with me as I worked to create the martini and mocktini recipes.

Many thanks to Liz Bacon Brownson of Oh! Creative (ohcreative-pdx.com), who is my trusted confidant. She has helped me keep my eye on the prize and stay focused so that I always stay true to my message and my brand.

To my husband, Ron Jaecks, who has supported me and encouraged me every step of the way. His love for me and belief in me has given me the freedom to pursue my dreams and to believe they can come true!

Finally, I want to thank all the women who listened to my messages, attended my events this past year, and truly became my tribe. Your enthusiasm for this project was an energy I turned to whenever I needed to push through and finish another step of the process. Thank you for believing in me and sharing with me your own journeys.

Table of Contents

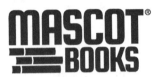

www.mascotbooks.com

Martinis & Menopause

This book is not intended as a substitute for the medical advice of physicians. The reader should regularly consult a physician in matters relating to his/her health and particularly with respect to any symptoms that may require diagnosis or medical attention.

For more information, please contact:
Mascot Books
620 Herndon Parkway, Suite 320
Herndon, VA 20170
info@mascotbooks.com

Library of Congress Control Number: 2018901081

CPSIA Code: PROPM0218A
ISBN-13: 978-1-68401-794-2

Printed in the United States

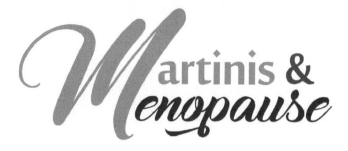

Martinis & Menopause

Strategies, Science,
and Sips that

Empower
Women

to Beat the
Hormone Groan

Kelli Jaecks

Introduction

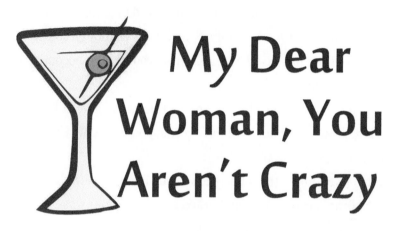

My Dear Woman, You Aren't Crazy

The Change is Real

Let's be real: our bodies change. Our hormones groan. Our relationships flux. Our priorities shift. And as Heraclitus said, "The only thing that is constant is change." Understanding what our bodies are going through and how to fully embrace this change while relieving its negative effects can bring you the knowledge and empowerment you need to not only live well, but to thrive. That's what this book is all about.

The truth is, most of the women who are going through menopause aren't talking about it. Instead, they suffer alone with the shame of their symptoms, fighting to just make it through the days as "normally" as possible. (Normal being how they felt before all these changes started happening.) Because, let's be honest: our grandmothers didn't talk about menopause, and our mothers didn't talk about it—if anything, it was a taboo subject, mentioned briefly and haltingly, creating a sense of shame around the entire topic.

It's time to talk about it.

Going through menopause can be compared to being taken hostage. Suddenly, your life is changed and it feels as though someone or something else has snatched it away from you. I call it becoming a Hormone Hostage.

Do you find yourself feeling and doing things you haven't before? Does it feel like your body is betraying you, and is just not behaving in the same ways as usual?

Perhaps you take others hostage in your home or work life with your scathing remarks, leaving burned corpses in your wake as you turn into a witch and lose all emotional control.

Or do you wake up multiple times a night with sweat running down all the cracks of your body, feeling like an insomniac hostage as your mind keeps whirring with all the stresses facing your day, week, and life?

Maybe your hostage situation involves seemingly non-stop, gushing periods, or surprise visits at the most unexpected (and least opportune) times.

Perhaps you're taken hostage by food cravings seemingly... Out. Of. Your. Control. Compelling you to finish that bag of chips, scarf down that leftover mac and cheese with bacon (after just finishing dinner), and drain that wine bottle. You feel crazy, knowing this isn't your rational self acting—your body feels suddenly possessed by a hungry, emotional, manic force with the hurricane-like power to blow through any snacks standing in your way.

My Dear Woman, You Aren't Crazy

Welcome to the Menopause Zone. You are going through 'The Change.' You are in perimenopause, or possibly well into menopause and sometimes when we get here, we just don't recognize ourselves. I get it. THIS is what I mean when I say: you are officially a Hormone Hostage.

It's time to break free.

The more we learn about menopause, share our own stories, and hear what others are going through, the more we normalize the conversation and bring the truth about ourselves into the light. What could be more exciting, empowering, and freeing than that?!

Some women will experience premature menopause (before the age of 40), through genetic reasons or medical intervention. Premature or early menopause may be induced through surgery, radiation, or chemotherapy. If this is the case, your body experiences a sudden drop in hormone levels, rather than the gradual, slow decline of natural menopause. Still, whether you travel through this stage early or take the usual route, the change is real. Either way, the strategies provided in this book can help you. Each of us is completely unique, so it's important to discover what strategies will work best to help our individual bodies transition gracefully and powerfully through menopause.

I find that so many women are confused and disempowered when it comes to this time of their life. Their hormones start whacking out, and they immediately feel like a prisoner on a downhill ride to somewhere they have no desire to go. But what would happen if we flipped this on its head, and became empowered and informed about these changes, so we could actually optimize our physical health, sensuality, and emotional world? Menopause is not only a vital change in every woman's life—it's an opportunity to embrace your womanhood and reignite your power.

No More Shame

Once a Hormone Hostage, I'm now a survivor who has lived through this entire transitional phase of my life, and am living happily on the other side—the side of freedom! The Hostage zone for me included most of the symptoms you'll read about in this book; I worked hard to understand what was happening inside of me and to find workable solutions to live better and feel better. I want to share what I learned with you, so you too can break free from the Hormone Hostage Zone.

As I journeyed through my own menopause transition, I started speaking to groups of women, teaching the Science of Why these things happen within our bodies, and providing helpful strategies to live as our best selves through it all. As I travelled all around the country, women would ask me, "What is happening to my body? What can I do to feel better?"

It's clear that women want pertinent information and practical solutions to the challenges they face during this part of their lives. For me, it was simply not okay to feel so out of control with regards to what was happening with my body, and I became determined to understand the truth and share it with women embarking on this journey.

But perhaps what's even worse than the disempowerment stemming from lack of knowledge about what's happening is the massive shame that so many women feel associated with their changing bodies. Sadly, many of us women in this transition phase feel a dislike, and even loathing, towards our bodies and how they are changing, from the embarrassment of having a hot flash in a public place, to projecting self-hate on our body as it packs on the pounds, to silencing ourselves when it comes to communicating our changing sexual needs. This shame has got to go! Going through menopause is not shameful, it's natural. The aging female body is not shameful, but a beautiful vessel for your growing wisdom and personal power. I want to empower you to live out loud, make choices to feel great about yourself, and own who you are as you age.

Knowledge is Power

Here in the 21st century, everything science and nerdy is trending—have you noticed? One of the easiest ways to stay young while aging is to know what's going on around you and shift with the times. It's cool to be "in the know," so get ready to geek out with the science that will empower you back into your body and health. (I'll make it easy, I promise!)

Black horn-rimmed glasses—check!
Girl-power in the boys' world—check!
Getting accolades and awards for KNOWING things that have nothing to do with your outward appearance—check!

First woman presidential candidate for a major political party of the United States—check!

The science behind female health is fascinating, and KNOWLEDGE is POWER! So, when your significant other says, "What? You're having your period again? Didn't you just go through that?" you can give an empowered reply:

"Why yes, I did just go through that, and the reason is that my reproductive system is beginning its journey to SHUTDOWN. My hormones are shifting, sometimes daily, so that's why I got my period again."

Isn't it great to be the smarty-pants who knows stuff? And when you know the Science of Why, you no longer feel like you're losing your mind or your grip on reality. On the contrary, you become strong and confident in your hormonal changes, knowing what to expect and how you can best work with that. And perhaps most importantly, you can better allow "grace through change" to be your mantra, rather than "anger and freak-out."

Think for a moment about the negative connotations our culture currently has of a menopausal woman. This time of life is often used as an excuse to be the witch, lashing out at coworkers and loved ones alike with negative, screaming accusations, or quietly seething with so much negative energy that no one wants to be around you.

Some women tend to shut themselves off from others, falling into depression over their various symptoms. Those around us are often walking on eggshells for fear of the hormonal explosion. Society has this idea that the menopausal woman is incredibly moody, unstable, and hard to be around. So not only do women feel they are a Hormone Hostage, but their loved ones do too.

Knowledge is the key to unlocking yourself from the hostage trap—but so many women never take the time to empower themselves, believing the science behind it all to be "over their head." In this book, we're going to blast this belief apart, making science sexy and accessible and empowering you with the knowledge you need to take back control of your life and feel great again.

Story. Sip. Science. Strategy.

While the journey of menopause may seem overwhelming, don't worry: we're going to break it all down into four easy steps every chapter.

Story – Each chapter will tell the story of a different woman going through her own unique journey while outlining one of the top ten symptoms experienced during menopause. Rather than trying to understand the science of menopause through some dry medical text, you'll get a real-life picture of what happens during menopause, and how the symptoms affect different people. You may even find a part of yourself in each woman's story as she shares the unique experience of menopause on her body, mind, and emotions.

Sip – At this point in each chapter, we'll take a quick break to mix up a martini or mocktini to prepare for the next stage of learning all the science and strategies to beat the Hormone Groan. Each chapter will feature recipes for you to try that relate to the story and symptom you've just read about. This is a time for you to sit down, relax, and take the stress off, as you contemplate what is happening to you and get ready to TAKE YOUR LIFE BACK.

Why am I talking about martinis in my book about menopause? Because, girlfriends, the journey we are on is not always easy or pleasant, and some of the science and news about what our bodies are going through can be tough to take. The lifestyle choices we often need to make in order to get through this transition gracefully are not always our first instinct—at times, you might feel like kicking the truth to the curb. But since we all must go through it, let's have some fun and laughter along the way!

The martini itself is a metaphor for sit down, relax, let's learn something and have a good time while doing it. Community is part of the martini experience too—sharing time with friends, encouraging one another, and seeing our changing bodies together, with a more positive, happier view. Supporting one another as we sip and share.

I am not advocating overindulgence, or alcoholism, or even alcohol for those who don't want it or can't have it. In fact, sharing a yummy mocktini or other non-alcoholic beverage can serve the same purpose! The martini as metaphor is open to any sort of beverage, shared with your wonderful self, or in a group of friends. The idea is to create and share drinks that are fun and yummy, can be shaken or stirred, and have infinite varieties—just like we, as women, are infinitely unique.

Shake, stir, and sip. Learning is empowering, and enjoying the journey is always recommended.

Science + Strategy – With martini or mocktini in hand, we will then dive into the Science of Why this is happening, explaining the physiology behind each symptom in plain English so you can become empowered with new knowledge and understanding. You'll get tons of practical tips and "news you can use" to live better. Finally, each chapter will end with actionable strategies to make positive changes for yourself during this transitional time.

Reading stories while learning about symptoms, sipping on delicious martinis and mocktinis, understanding the Science of Why, and discovering useful strategies will help you beat the Hormone Groan and take back your life—so you can once again be living as your sexy, savvy, most powerful self.

Sound good? Let's do this!

Fantastic Four

There are four overarching, superhero strategies that will help you navigate every one of the symptoms of menopause. In fact, any woman of any age will benefit by getting a jump on these. They are found in the appendix in the back of the book, but I refer to them in almost every chapter. They are exercise, food choices, hormone replacement therapy, and sleep. As you read through the chapters, please thumb back and use this appendix as further fuel for you to make positive changes for your health.

Definitions

Remember having to learn the language of texts with shortened versions of words and acronyms like LOL, LMAO, and BFF? Knowing the definitions of things helps immensely in getting on the same page with what we're talking about. You already know what you've been feeling and experiencing, so let's put some terminology to it all so we can speak the same language.

Here are the basic definitions you'll need as you read on:

Perimenopause - This is the space all women pass through on their way to full menopause and life after periods. Your body is shutting down the reproductive zone, biologically changing from having the ability to procreate. That's a good thing—I for one, would not want to have the ability to get pregnant my whole life. Thank you, perimenopause! Sometimes called pre-menopause, these changes usually begin to happen somewhere in the early to mid-forties, with symptoms showing up in various ways and to varying degrees. Each body passes through perimenopause a little bit differently, depending on many factors like genetics and lifestyle. Perimenopause and menopause are normal states of natural aging, so don't worry or freak out when you reach this phase of life. If anything, it shows that your body is jiving along in its normal cycles. Perimenopause can last anywhere from two to ten years, so buckle up for the ride!

Menopause - We often hear a woman say, "I am going through menopause." However, menopause itself is only one day. Menopause is the day you haven't had a period for 12 months in a row. Period.

So, a woman is not literally in menopause when she speaks about it, but is either perimenopausal or postmenopausal. However, in our everyday language we often say things like, "I am in menopause," "I'm menopausal," or "I am going through menopause." All of these phrases are referring to the sometimes crazy changes we go through during perimenopause on our way to that magical day when we reach menopause. However, in our culture and daily vernacular, we usually just use "menopause" to describe the phase we are going through, and that's all good. We don't want to get hung up on the words, I just want you to have clarity.

The average age of a woman reaching menopause is 51 years. You may reach this stage earlier or later, but each journey is as different and unique as you are. Embrace yours!

Post-menopause - Technically, post-menopause is all the days AFTER the day you haven't had a period for 12 straight months. You can shout Hallelujah! When you finally get there. A whole new part of your fabulous life will open up.

Okay, now that we have the definitions out of the way, we have an understanding of what we're really talking about and can move forward, on the same page.

Signs and Symptoms of Perimenopause

I'm going to be real with you: the journey through perimenopause is rife with symptoms that, if you're not aware of what's happening, can leave you feeling crazy and confused in your body. Luckily, we're going to go through the top ten symptoms so you know what to expect and how to best deal with them.

The hormonal fluctuations happening during perimenopause can affect vasomotor, cognitive, vulva-vaginal (What? Yes, that is really a word, and the correct medical term for the entire clitoris-labia-vagina area of our bodies), skeletal, and dental systems within the female body. It's no wonder that many women are overwhelmed by their bodily changes and feel at a loss as to how to manage them.

During perimenopause and up until menopause, the ovaries are gradually shutting down, making less of the hormones estrogen and progesterone. Hormonal levels can be highly erratic, exhibiting differing fluctuation patterns from month to month, even hour to hour. The changing levels of these hormones are what trigger perimenopausal symptoms.

Symptoms can include, but are not limited to:

- Changes in the pattern of your periods
- Either longer or shorter time span in-between and/or lighter or heavier flow
- Hot flashes
- Night sweats
- Mood swings
- Mental fog
- Change in sexual desire
- Bone loss
- Depression and sadness
- Extreme irritability
- Strong food cravings

These signs and symptoms can range from annoying to debilitating. But having a road map of what to expect can help, as you can see what's coming and attribute these changes to normal hormone fluctuations, rather than some insidious health problem or mental disorder.

Welcome to discovery—may you be empowered to beat the Hormone Groan, and escape the chains of the Hormone Hostage.

Freedom to live your best self—"Go Meno!"

– Kelli

Chapter One

Brain Fog

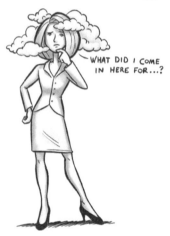

Meet Aimee

Aimee is an accomplished professional in the sales industry, a real go-getter. She has a reputation for razor-sharp intellect coupled with a flair for knowing how to close any deal. A true extrovert, Aimee relishes the thrill of working a room for her next successful contact. She is hardwired to spin many plates in the air at once—and make dinner while she's at it. Recently, however, something has changed. Aimee turned 45 and is experiencing peri-menopausal brain fog.

Story

Hello, my name is Aimee and I am proud to say that I am the Vice President of Sales at a large, high-tech software company. Recently, I heard that I am on the short list for the next promotion to National Division Manager, which is exciting because not only does this position usually go to a man, but I would be the youngest person to get this title in the history of our company!

However, I've got a secret that I'm hiding. Lately, I have been experiencing episodes where my brain simply turns to mush and it is affecting my work. There are multiple times throughout the day when I simply cannot focus. I find myself saying things that I have NEVER said before: Where are my glasses? It's on the tip of my tongue... Did I turn off the coffee pot? I mean, really! Am I losing my mind?

Often it feels like I am moving through a thick, soupy fog. When the fog won't lift, I get up, I walk the floor, I take deep breaths, I get a cup of tea. I try anything to clear the haze in my head. Sometimes these tactics work, but sometimes they don't; more and more I am getting seriously behind on my daily goals and weekly reports. I have always taken pride in my efficiency, and I feel like, for the first time in my life, I can't meet my own standards.

I am both annoyed and really, really scared.

Take yesterday, for instance. My boss asked me for the data report on a large deal that had just closed. I was the lead on this project and knew the details of it inside and out.

Well, usually.

"Aimee, the report?" he asked.

My. Mind. Went. Blank. I couldn't even remember the name of

the damn company! I panicked for a few seconds, and then tried to distract him by asking about his golf game. I knew he would go on and on about it, and, as usual, I was right. As I pretended to listen to him brag on, I began frantically combing through documents in my computer, hoping to provoke my memory to recall whatever the hell it was he had asked for! Mercifully, I happened upon a document that brought me back to my brain. Just as he was ending the enthralling story of the hole-in-one he had scored, I chimed in, congratulated his amazing golf success, and confirmed the report I would soon be sending over to him. Whew! That was close!

You see, it is not uncommon in this new universe I now live in to barely escape bad situations. I seem to be constantly asking people if they have seen my cell phone. Just yesterday, my daughter called to see why I hadn't picked her up from her Tuesday play rehearsal. Why hadn't I? Because I was thinking it was MONDAY. As I sped to the school to get my grumpy teenager, I began to really worry. What is going on with me? Why can't I remember even the simplest things? I have got to figure this out, or I'll be saying good-bye to my fancy promotion, and hello to an eternally grumpy teenager.

Sip

Hormone Happy Hour

Do Aimee's symptoms resonate with you? Perhaps you see yourself in similar situations and internal conflicts, wondering just where your brain went. It's time to sit down with a big, electrifying, brain opening martini, or brain calming mocktini, and ponder what's been going on.

While you and Aimee are considering your brain function, break out the absinthe. Not sure what that is? Absinthe has a storied history; often called "The Green Fairy," it is believed to have mild hallucinogenic properties, a wonderful alcohol to deal with brain fog! Also, it has been imbibed by some of the most creative and intelligent folks in our history including Ernest Hemingway, James Joyce, Pablo Picasso, and Vincent Van Gogh—giants who clearly needed optimal brain function for their arts. Unfortunately, no women pop up on the most famous absinthe drinkers list—let's change that!

Dream On Martini

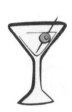

2 oz vodka or gin
½ oz dry vermouth
3 oz root beer
A few drops of absinthe
One piece black licorice

Take your martini glass, pour two to three drops of absinthe into it, and swirl the glass around. Put the alcohols into a shaker with ice, shake vigorously, and pour into the prepared glass. Add the root beer. Garnish with the licorice stick.

Dream On Mocktini

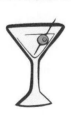

5 oz root beer
2 oz licorice flavoring
Two pieces black licorice

Grate one piece of licorice into glass, using the smallest grate size. Fill glass with ice. Pour in root beer and licorice flavoring. Garnish with remaining licorice stick.

The health properties of licorice include lifting your mood and calming your anxiety. Perfect. Your brain should now be sufficiently flying.

Science of Why

Now that we have a delicious libation in hand, it's time to bring some understanding to why Aimee's brain seems to be cutting out at the most inopportune times and losing its connection to mission control.

"Drop it like it's hot"

While this phrase refers to a dance move involving strong thigh and glute muscles, thus being able to "drop it" (your beautiful behind) and then get back up while gyrating and grooving to the tunes, I'm referring here to dropping dopamine levels throughout the day. This is the most likely culprit contributing to Aimee's lack of concentration and fuzzy brain.

During perimenopause, the hormones are waxing and waning, surging and retreating, shooting all over the place. Your brain is very sensitive to hormonal changes, and it is the engine driving many of the symptoms' train. Both the estrogen and testosterone hormones affect neurotransmitters, specifically those that affect much of our mood and memory. Diminishing levels of hormones means diminishing levels of neurotransmitters. So those specific cars on the brain train are waiting for the hormonal "hook-up" to bring them along the tracks. When there are not enough hormones, there will be no hook-up, and no firing of these neurotransmitters, leaving you in a fog (1). All making sense so far?

Now, a closer look at these neurotransmitters and their disappearing act. You've probably heard of them: norepinephrine, dopamine, and serotonin. All of these neurotransmitters vitally affect our moods, energy levels, and emotional states. A drop in dopamine specifically can cause a lapse in concentration (brain fog), and we need stable estrogen levels to maintain a stable mood and focus. So, the combined diminishment of estrogen and dopamine in the body and brain amplifies the frustrating haziness that descends upon your brain during perimenopause (2).Like San Francisco in the spring, you are enshrouded in fog.

The good news is, a recent study found that the mental challenges of a foggy brain and loss of concentration are usually only temporary in the perimenopausal woman, and some of us may not experience this at all. A large study of over 2000 women published in 2017 concludes that if women suffer from Brain Fog, or more scientifically stated, "cognitive decline," during midlife, this does not foretell more decline later in life (3). So, pick up that martini and celebrate, because it's just a transitional phenomenon. You aren't losing your mind—well, you kind of are, but only temporarily (4). Cheers!

Strategy

Tips for living your best self

Brain fog begone! To see things clearly and get our brains working fabulously for us, check out these tips:

Tip #1: Brain health

It's no secret we need to keep challenging our brain, helping it function at the top of its game throughout our life. There are entire books written about the brain, brain science, and brain health which you can go read if you so choose. Many of these books offer actionable strategies and exercises for keeping your brain sharp and on point. One of my favorites is *The Female Brain* by Louann Brizendine, M.D. (5).

But for now, here's a quick down-and-dirty list to get you started:

Learn something new – New languages, musical instruments, words to a favorite song, tap dancing, a new knitting technique... this world is chock-full of cool and interesting things to learn. Consider yourself a lifelong learner, and your brain will stay in its best possible shape throughout your time on this planet. Stay curious, and take advantage of new situations and opportunities that come into your life. For example, my new son-in-law is Brazilian, and he and my daughter speak fluent Portuguese together. I'm thinking that as a lifelong learner, I'd better start studying my Portuguese. One day they may have children, and I'd love to be able to communicate with them in that language. Learning new things can open up doors and expose you to different opportunities or groups of people that enrich your life. Several years ago, I decided to take voice (singing) lessons. I liked theatre and thought I would try my hand at being in a musical. So, I sought out a voice teacher who specializes in musical theater, rather than classical music. I have been with her for eight years now, off and on as my schedule allows, and have been a lead actor/singer in multiple productions. Talk about the joy of being exposed to a whole new community of loving, fun, accepting people! My life has been enriched beyond what I could imagine, all because I chose to learn a new skill. And just think of all the new nerve endings that have been created in my healthier brain! You may not want to sing and act in front of large groups of people, but learning something new that interests you will absolutely enrich your life and brain.

Social networking – Now, before you run away screaming that you hate networking, hear me out. Social connectivity with other humans is soooo good for our brains. Your mind is constantly processing what each person looks like, matching name to face, remembering facts about them, and making connections between people, flooding your brain with feel-good endorphins from all that great connection—all great for brain health. Who doesn't love all that good, happy serotonin firing around when you're hanging out with people you love? Expanding your business or social contacts, being involved in groups, large or small, and being with people whose energy you enjoy and thrive on all work to blow away the brain fog and leave your head clearer.

Feel-good activities – What smells good to you? What feels good on your skin? Is there a place in your home or workplace that makes you feel calm when you see it or walk by? What sounds make you happy? What music soothes your soul? Activate your senses each day to stimulate your brain power. Exercise comes in here as well, as a way to reach that endorphin high as you break through to sweating. And yes, even sex counts as a feel-good activity—it is indeed great for your brain.

Tip #2: Find a good acupuncturist

It can be difficult to fully understand how acupuncture works if you haven't been exposed to it or had training in the practice. But as a therapy for perimenopause, it works beautifully. Basically, when you're highly stressed (as many of us are with the multiple responsibilities, activities, and obligations we face daily), you feel tense and your body tightens up. In Chinese medicine, your life energy is called "Qi," and when stressed, your Qi stagnates and does not circulate properly through your bloodstream. Stagnated Qi caused by stress leads our emotions to be affected with mood swings, irritability, and depression (to name just a few.) Deficient Qi also increases brain fog, as the brain is malnourished by a lack of vital, rich blood flow. When Qi is unblocked and released throughout the body through practices like acupuncture, perimenopause symptoms can be reduced and/or eliminated and your life energy can flow again.

I saw a highly trained, compassionate acupuncturist (she actually was a Western-trained MD with a Chinese doctorate in Acupuncture) for about six years while I was experiencing the worst of my perimenopausal symptoms. An acupuncture session puts you into such a deep state of relaxation; I would come out of the session feeling balanced and almost high. The cumulative effects over time helped elevate my mood, energy, and hormone balance, and I was able to beat the Hormone Groan.

The Fantastic Four have an important part to play in dispersing brain fog, so don't forget them. There are simple steps you can take in each of the Four Superhero strategies that will assist you in feeling better. Turn to the appendix now and take a look if you haven't already. Consistent vigorous exercise and hormone balance will help sharpen your mind and clear out the fog. The physical functioning of the brain itself will be enhanced by taking your Omega 3s, and getting enough sleep is needed to rest and recharge.

Take Action

- **Make a 5-Senses Happiness List of your own.** Think of what sights, sounds, smells, tastes, and touches bring you pleasure and write them down. Once you make your list, hang it where you can see it every day.
- **Get yourself out there!** What will you do this week to network with others? It can be business meetings, social get-togethers, your place of worship, a civic group, or perhaps volunteering in your community. Put a time and day in your weekly calendar to connect with others.
- **Dream a little.** What is something new you would like to do or try in the next three months? Do a little exploration into what you would need to do to get started. Buy supplies? Find a class? Tap into YouTube how-to videos? Then craft a plan and move towards making that dream of learning something new come true.

The Brain Fog Zone does not have to define you. While it is frustrating to constantly forget things and feel like you are losing your mental control, be kind and patient with yourself. There are many small (but profound) actions you can take to help with the brain fog phenomenon. Just know that this is transitional, and the more you work and stretch your brain, the easier it will be. Brain fog begone!

Chapter Two
The Bitch!

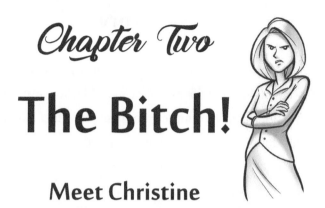

Meet Christine

Christine is cranky. You may have met Christine when she was in line behind you at the grocery store pointing out that you and your 17 items should NOT be in the 15 item Express Lane. She simply doesn't like chaos or rule breakers and she thrives on order and control. She hasn't always been like this, but recently she feels overwhelmed by her changing body, and keeps finding herself being taken hostage by her hormones. These things find her behaving like an out-and-out, no holds barred, complete and total...

B-I-T-C-H.

We all know the word. And none of us like being called it. Originally, the word bitch comes from the word bicche, which was developed from the Old English word bicce, and possibly derived from the Old Norse word bikkja, all meaning "female dog."

The term was first used as a disparaging insult against women sometime around the 15th century. No wonder we don't like it.

In today's world, when women are working so hard for the respect we deserve, I honestly don't advocate that you use it. However, Christine and I will use the word today, for this chapter. But only to make a point.

Story

Hi, I'm Christine and I lose my s*it when people don't do what they're supposed to do. I imagine a world where everyone pulls their own weight, and you can rely on them, but I feel like that world just simply doesn't exist. I have high standards. These expectations exist for everyone, including myself.

I've always been someone who likes to have order; some people call me a perfectionist. If that means I like to have things in their place, and everyone doing their job—what they are supposed to be doing—then fine, I'm a perfectionist.

I'm a paralegal, and work in a small office with one attorney, an administrative assistant, and a front office manager. My job is to help people get documents ready for their court dates, interface directly with—

Will you please STOP talking so loud on your cell phone? I am trying to have a conversation here, too! Good gracious!

Now where was I... oh yes... work. You see, I like to think my co-workers and I have pretty good relationships and, except for the boss, I consider them my friends. We often run out to catch a bite to eat together, and we seem to usually work in sync to keep the office flowing nicely. I generally get along well with all of them. This last year though? Not so much. They just haven't been doing ANYTHING right.

Take yesterday as an example. One of the files I needed for that day was not completed on time by our admin. And I just flipped out. I yelled at her, and as I yelled, I slammed the file drawer closed so hard it bounced back open. It was a serious rage-fest. I paused to get myself back under control, but the damage had already been done. I apologized, but she continues to keep her distance from me. I suppose I can't blame her.

I guess I find myself apologizing a lot lately. Not only at work, but at home, too.

Last weekend, I was so annoyed by everything, and by nothing. I can't really tell you why, but everything my husband said to me prompted a nasty, short, insulting response. It was like everything that came out of my mouth was ugly and hurtful. It was a good thing the kids were away at their grandparents' or they would have certainly been in the crossfire of all my negative torrents. Finally, by Sunday night, I began to wonder if my mood swings were possibly hormonal, and went to talk about it, calmly this time, to my husband. The poor guy seemed glad I was back. After a weekend of me snapping at him, I am sure he was tired of it. I said, "This is not about you. I am not even upset at you. This is about me and my changing, raging hormones. I'm sorry, please don't take it personally. I need you and your love and support to get through this."

Wow! He responded by giving me one of his great big bear hugs. That seemed to shift the tide and we could finally relax and enjoy the last couple of hours of the weekend before the kids came home.

But it's not fixed, yet. This whole "becoming the complete bitch" in 0-5 seconds is exhausting! And not surprisingly, I feel terrible, because my family, friends, and coworkers now see me as this raging, hostile person. I seem to be leaving charred hearts in my wake. It's not good.

I need some relief.

Sip

Hormone Happy Hour

Christine, shake it up and sit down with a Zen-Zone Martini or Mocktini. Lavender is known for its relaxation properties, something anyone experiencing this hormone zone needs. Let the relaxation begin as we discover just what is going on and what we can do about it.

Zen-Zone Martini

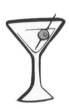

2 oz vanilla vodka
½ fresh lemon, juiced
½ oz lavender syrup
1 sprig fresh lavender

Place all liquids in a shaker with ice. Shake vigorously. Strain into a chilled martini glass. Garnish with the lavender sprig.

Zen-Zone Mocktini

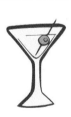

3 oz soda water or lemon-lime soda
½ fresh lemon, juiced
½ oz lavender syrup
2-3 drops vanilla extract to taste
1 sprig fresh lavender

Place all liquids in a shaker with ice. Stir vigorously. Strain into a chilled martini glass. Garnish with the lavender sprig.

Sip, smell, taste, feel the drink move down your throat, and into your stomach. Breathe deep. RELAX.

Science of Why

Does Christine's story sound familiar? There's a reason Christine turns into Godzilla and it's not because she wants to destroy those around her. Just as with brain fog, the culprit is waxing and waning hormone levels and brain chemistry caused by perimenopause or menopause. What you may not know is WHY the fluctuation of Christine's hormones transform her into the She Devil of Washington County.

Your emotions are highly connected to your brain chemistry. The brain's role in regulating mood and emotion is complex. But one thing we do know is that getting more of those calming and "feel good" neurotransmitters like serotonin is very important for emotion regulation. Serotonin is credited with affecting either directly or indirectly almost all of the cells within our brain. Its job is to enable and assist with communication of messages between brain cells. Because of this widespread influence, serotonin is thought to affect many symptoms and systems within the body including our mood, emotions, temperature regulation (hot flash), appetite, and sex drive.

In addition to all of this, lifestyle and certain medical changes can trigger irrational emotions. Lack of exercise, a poor diet of fast and processed foods, high consumption of caffeine, alcohol, sugars, and drugs (prescribed or not), and general stress that happens at mid-life can all contribute to the crazy emotional mood swings of the bitch symptoms. What? No wonder you feel like offing somebody.

Another big chunk of this Science of Why in relation to emotional health and balance has to do with your gut and digestion. The brain, your emotions, and your gut are intricately related to one another (1). Think about it: if you are sad or upset and start to cry, the physical impulse starts in your throat. It tightens up, you may have to swallow to stop the tears. This is an example of one part of your digestive tract, the upper GI and esophagus, responding physically to your emotions. Or when you are scared and highly nervous. Perhaps you must do a presentation at work in front of your boss and co-workers, and you feel it in your guts, you may get diarrhea or feel nauseated and have to excuse yourself to the restroom. That is another example of the gut and emotional brain responding to each other.

Why is your GI tract so connected to your emotions?

Because your gut actually has more nerve endings than your real brain and spinal cord combined. (WHO KNEW?) The ten-dollar medical term is the "Enteric Nervous System," but we commonly refer to this as, "The Little Brain". This enteric—read intestinal—nervous system provides more serotonin to your body than what we ordinarily think of as our nervous system. The serotonin produced by the Little Brain in your gut communicates with the brain in your head to create and release more serotonin. Bring on the double-whammy of feel-good-WOW.

So, if you want to stay sane on most days, pay attention to your digestive track. If you keep it healthy and working well, you'll have more of that glorious serotonin to keep you emotionally strong and stable.

Great! So, how do we get more emotional grounding, a healthier gut, and the feel-good substances flowing and working in the body? How do we live in a way that doesn't leave burned, emotionally-fried corpses in our wake?

Strategy

Tips for living your best self
Tip #1: Consider an OTC Phyto-Progesterone cream.

Phyto substances are made from plants and act as progesterone would in the body, filling up the hormone receptors. Most products are made from the wild yam plant and then converted to progesterone in the body. These are considered bio-identical, as the molecular structure is identical to the hormones our bodies manufacture. A progesterone cream is absorbed very well through the skin, and is recommended to rub onto areas of the body that have thinner skin such as the wrists, upper chest, neck, inner arms, and the palms of the hands and feet. It is then circulated throughout the body and able to fill the progesterone receptors.

Progesterone creams can help alleviate becoming the Bitch by helping to balance the emotions and taking off the irritation edge. When women come to me with this symptom, I recommend phyto-progesterones as the first line of defense. My favorite company is Emerita Pro-Gest. It's easy to get, easy to use, and totally takes the edge off, helping us ease out of the bitch zone (2).

Tip #2: Positive self-talk

Check your self-talk. We women are notorious for letting negative phrases about ourselves affect our emotional state—taking us into the Bitch Zone. How often do you get caught on a negative loop like this? "I am so fat and bloated today," "I look awful," "I can't do this, it's too much," "I'll never be as good as..." "I hate her," "Why can't they just do their job?!" "My hair is so... frizzy, greasy, stringy, puffy, flat, thin, curly, ugly..." "These pants make me look fat," "Why would anyone want to hang out with me?"

You get the picture; I bet you could write your own chapter on the negative self-talk that you personally listen to over time. STOP IT! Whatever you tell yourself, about yourself, is what you will be—as your words become a self-fulfilling prophecy. If you change the conversation in your head, your attitude and emotions will change.

I recommend a book by Jennifer Powers, called *Oh Shift*, which is an excellent guide to help you shift your inner conversation and help turn negatives into positives (3).

If you are engaging in positive self-talk like:

"I'm going to have a great day,"

"I am confident and powerful,"

"I can handle anything that comes my way today with calm and grace,"

I guarantee you will have a better day. Positive self-talk works to re-wire your brain map activity. There is an entire science on affirmations and putting positive thoughts and energy out into the universe, and I'm telling you, if you engage in that, you will be happier and live with less negative emotions.

Your episodes of rage and bitchy irritability will diminish. Try it!

Tip # 3: Tune into your senses

Anything that brings you calm and pleasure will also help with irritability and release more serotonin into your brain. The same neuropathways that light up with pleasure and send your dopamine soring to reduce brain fog also serve as serotonin enhancers to calm the raging beast.

When you are upset, can you get to a physical space that makes you feel better? A quiet courtyard at work, your favorite chair in your home, a beautiful lake or shoreline? What is pleasing to you? The sound of a river running over the rocks? The ocean waves washing onshore and swishing through the sand on their way out? Birds chirping and trilling? Symphonies playing? A certain scented candle? The feel of a cozy blanket? The beauty of the brain is, even if you can't be with these places or things physically, you can simply close your eyes and picture them, take deep calming breaths, and be there in your mind.

Pay attention to the sights, sounds, and smells that bring you pleasure, and get more of that in your life. I have a large set of chimes outside my front door, and they are in the key of "C." If I am having a particularly bad, bitchy day, where the negativity and irritation wants to take me over, I will go outside my front door and lightly touch them, (or bang them together! Argggggghhhh!) and the chimes will sound out. Whenever I hear these chimes, I immediately relax, and feel a sense of serenity and peace. I simply LOVE the sound they make. I can stand still in that moment, listening and breathing deeply with a smile in my soul.

Try to populate your everyday world with things that delight the senses and make you feel happy. It will definitely help with those feelings of intense irritation and irrational anger, saving you and your loved ones from the Hormone Groan.

Another sensory help in beating the Bitch back is meditation. The act of focusing on your breath, working to clear your mind of distractions and stressors, will actually make your mind more calm and focused. Meditation can be done in five to ten minutes; it doesn't have to be a long, quiet time. Some find it productive to meditate upon waking in the morning, setting their mind to the positive before the day gets going. I personally use meditation to end my day, letting go of any negative thoughts or actions that I perceived from others, or that I partook in, and letting go of any disappointments I had with myself or others. I let the negative go, breathing it out, and focus on gratitude, rest, and envisioning all good things for the next day ahead. It only takes a few minutes, and I am reset to calm and peace. There are many books, resources, and websites to help you get started in this simple practice (4).

Tip #4: Gut health

What you eat is so important to feeling good emotionally. That Little Brain in your gut wants to be firing on all cylinders so you can optimize the feel-good substances running through your veins and be more stable emotionally. Playing detective to figure out how you are feeling when you eat certain foods is a positive step to emotional health and brain clarity. If you suspect, for example, that milk and milk products affect your gut negatively (like when you eat a big ole bowl of decadent ice-cream, and then get gas and diarrhea), then perhaps try an elimination diet, where you cut out all milk products for a couple of weeks and see if your symptoms abate, and you feel better. You then add those types of foods back into your diet, one by one, and can determine how they affect you.

Fast food and highly processed foods also negatively affect your gut health. They are chock-full of extra sugars, salts, and chemicals, with many of the vitamins and nutrients removed from the original food source. Add in whatever antibiotics and fertilizers are used to grow your grains, vegetables, and animals for meat, and you have very unhealthy "food" being chewed, chomped, swallowed, and massaged through your GI tract. When you are on a constant diet of these types of foods, the healthy gut bacteria get destroyed, and these processed substances serve as fertilizer for the bad, disease-causing bacteria. Oh, and they feed the yeast that may be in there too. NOT GOOD. Women in particular are susceptible to yeast infections, and they generally start right here in our gut. And think about that—if you have a yeast infection, or any GI upset and disturbance, you generally do not feel upbeat, happy, or positive. Work to cut out the foods that make you unwell, and make simple steps to buy, cook, and eat foods that support your physical and mental health.

The tips to a healthy gut are further outlined in the Fantastic Four section. Flip to the back of the book now and check it out.

Take Action

- **Take inventory of what's in those cupboards.** It might be time to go grocery shopping. Make a plan for eating so you are less tempted by your busy life to rely on fast food as a regular meal source. Be brave, throw away the processed foods you find in your cupboards, and replace them with organic, whole foods.

- **Check your self-talk.** For two days, pay attention to the kinds of messages you are allowing to run through your brain. Note when they are negative towards yourself, or the circumstances you find yourself in. Shift your thinking. Work to tell yourself positive affirming messages. Be your own best friend.

- **Revisit your five senses happiness list.** And make time to experience them this week. Find a quiet five minutes in your day to simply close your eyes and breathe in and out deeply, focusing on your breath.

The Bitch Zone does not have to define you! Now that you've got a better understanding of why your brain and emotions want to respond this way, and have some tools in your tool kit on how to alleviate some of that, you're ready to Zen out, put some new strategies into action, and beat the Hormone Groan.

Chapter Three

Basement Blues

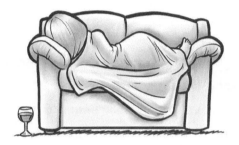

Meet Elaine

Elaine is a doting mom, a happy wife, and a successful small business owner. The oldest of 7, her gentle, open nature makes it easy for her siblings and friends to seek Elaine out for advice and she gives it, gladly. The glass has always been half-full from Elaine's perspective, and she works hard to keep her life in balance and her family happy. Steady and stable-minded, Elaine generally laughs easily and has a kind word for everyone. Lately though, she finds herself feeling more than a little blue.

Story

Hi, I'm Elaine. I am the owner of a successful online jewelry business, the mother of twin twelve-year-old girls, and wife to my amazing husband, Jeffrey. I love my family, and my work is satisfying and creative. All this is usually enough to make me smile, but lately I feel things changing.

This morning, after dropping my girls off at school, I feel myself becoming annoyed with how bright the sun is shining. I trudge home, and... sit. Even now, looking around at my kitchen, with its half-filled cereal bowls, butter knives covered in peanut butter, jam jars opened and still out, I correctly survey that it is, indeed, a mess.

But, I just can't.

It is all too much for me today. Thank goodness, I have drapes that keep out all that light. I feel like I'm slowly sinking in quicksand. It's so hard to move or even breathe. Thoughts slowly fill my head.

"Elaine. Pull yourself together," I say out loud. I try and find the strength to put things away. I stand at the counter and do nothing.

I should work. I should clean. I should shower, I think to myself. I should. I should. I should. I head to my bedroom, crawl back under the covers, and I don't.

Ordinarily, I enjoy these hours in my day when my man is at his job, the kids are at school, and I have time to work on my business and do some household chores. I'm certainly not perfect, nor is my house. I'm more artist than housecleaner and, even at my best, I believe that if there is love in the home, then a few piles of dirty clothes and some unopened junk mail doesn't matter.

Why am I feeling like this? I think back to when I turned 44. It was around that birthday that I began to experience waves of sadness and depression, for no real reason at all. Some days, I just cry. Those are the days—like today—that I come home from dropping off the kids, turn off my phone, close the drapes, and crawl back in bed. I do nothing, I accomplish nothing. It feels just awful.

Occasionally, though less and less these days, I can snap out of it and shake it off. More and more, however, I find myself almost unable to keep it from my family. When the kids squabble, or if my husband so much as looks at me the wrong way, I retreat to the bathroom, so they don't have to see me cry.

Last weekend, my husband held my hands and asked me what he could do to help. I love him so much, and I know that he and our children aren't the reason for these blues. I used to be such a different person. I miss the goofy fun I once had, and want to figure out what I need to do to find my smile again.

Sip

Hormone Happy Hour

Elaine needs some relief, some understanding of what is happening to her, and some concrete strategies to get out of the Basement Blues. Let's join her in taking our focus off these symptoms, and onto something more fun: a party-themed martini and mocktini! Collect your ingredients and get ready to shake it up! This drink is sure to bring the happy back.

Party Hearty Martini

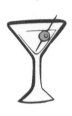

2 oz vodka
½ oz crème de violet liquour
½ oz cranberry juice
Splash of soda water
Cake decorating sprinkles

Rim top of glass with cranberry juice, tip upside down into a plate of cake sprinkles. Shake alcohols and juice vigorously, pour into the party glass, and top with soda.

Party Hearty Mocktini

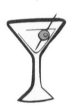

2 oz soda water or lemon-lime soda
½ oz violet flavoring
½ oz cranberry juice
Cake decorating sprinkles

Rim top of glass with cranberry juice, tip upside down into a plate of cake sprinkles. Pour cranberry juice and soda into shaker, stir, and pour into the party glass.

Science of Why

Now that you've stirred up your pretty little libation, let's learn what's going on and how to shake off the Blues. To understand these emotional downturns, including the anxiety levels and all the crying, we look again at the brain, hormone levels, and what might be happening in your life circumstances to bring you down and keep you in the Emotional Basement.

Here is a partial list of symptoms you may experience in the Basement, or this season sometimes called the "Menopause Blues." Can I get a country song here?!

- You no longer get pleasure from activities that used to make you happy
- Change in your sleep patterns, see the chapter on night sweats—leading to fatigue and loss of energy
- Feelings of worthlessness, guilt, or sadness
- Crying for no reason at all
- Being irritable or agitated most of the time

Any of this resonate with you?

Brain Chemistry

No surprise here, one answer to the Science of Why is—you guessed it—the brain chemistry itself. It is reported that lower estrogen levels may have some effect on perimenopausal depression, but it is not a key player. (Yes, you read that right. Estrogen is not the culprit here.) Rather, the lowering of estrogens and progesterones trigger a different brain chemical to increase, called Monoamine Oxidase, or MAO-A. Hang with me here—this is a King Kong chemical.

Research shows that as key estrogens lower, MAO-A rises, like King Kong towering above the buildings of New York. The result is that the MAO-A becomes a denser, thicker, more menacing molecule, and basically eats up your feel-good neurotransmitters in the brain like serotonin, norepinephrine, and dopamine. With lower levels of these three, your moods become un-stable, leading to depressive feelings and symptoms (1). Watch out world—the Hormone Hostage Zone has arrived!

Interestingly, research shows this MAO-A action is also a key contributor to post-partum depression, a time after childbirth when women's hormone levels are also trying to reach equilibrium. For us women, we experience fluctuating hormones in every stage of life, from reproduction to post-menopause. The symptoms are real, the feelings are real, and the struggle to stay balanced is real.

Women in the transitional menopausal place are four times more likely to develop depressive symptoms and two times more likely to develop full blown clinical depression than women who are not in this time of life (2).

Ack! Kelli, give me some good news, I'm drowning in the negative here. OK, but before we get to the important tips on HOW TO FEEL BETTER, please do some self-assessment.

It can be difficult to differentiate whether you are experiencing full blown clinical depression, episodic depression brought on by outside events, or depressive feelings brought on by perimenopause. A good rule of thumb is to know that if you feel depressed continuously for two weeks or longer, it's time to make an appointment with your health care provider and get to the bottom of it. If your depression comes and goes, lasting only a few days at a time, you can safely assume it's those pesky Menopausal Blues brain chemicals all worked up by fluctuating hormones. Either way, there's no reason to suffer for more than a few days without seeking relief.

Keep in mind that events such as divorce, aging and sick parents, job loss, or a partner's failing health can trigger sadness during this time of life. Additional factors that may contribute to Basement Blues are low self-esteem, a negative view of your aging and your changing body (Please, we all deal with this!) and sleep deprivation. Pair these with hormonal imbalances and the usual ill-health culprits of smoking, sedentary lifestyle, too much alcohol, or processed foods – and you've got triggers that can push you over the edge of depression.

Fortunately, there are things you can do every day to take down the King Kong trying to crush you! Read on to learn what you can do to help yourself through it.

Strategy

Tips for living your best self
Tip #1: Self-care and self-love

It is so important to carve out time for doing things that you love and bring a smile to your face. It is not selfish to love yourself and do things that bring you pleasure—in fact, it's necessary for your health. I know that self-love can be an overwhelming topic, but it is so necessary to get to that place where you like yourself, you accept yourself, and you love yourself.

When fighting the Menopause Blues, make the effort to do the little things that bring light into your day. Do you love to soak in a hot bath? Then do that. Take a warm bath with lavender salts, and feel the stress melting away from your arms, legs, and chest. Let the water embrace you and dissolve all the negative feelings away.

Do you take time to get your needs met, rather than only living to meet the needs of others? It is easier to set priorities for taking care of yourself when you are not feeling down or blue, but the fact is, you need to take excellent care of yourself if you want to take care of others in your life.

What is it you need each day? I know I need quiet time in the morning, just for myself, to wake up slowly, meditate on the day ahead, set my top three tasks I need to get done that day, and generally to reconnect with myself, my soul. To make this happen, I make the choice to get up 40 minutes earlier than necessary, every day. Whether I am at home or travelling, I build in that quiet alone time I need each day. The benefits of this practice far outweigh the extra minutes of sleep.

Another strategy for developing self-love is to be your own best friend. What kind of positive things would your best friend have to say about you? They would not be saying negative things to pull you down (if you have those kinds of friends, they are doing you no good). So, talk to yourself the way your best friend would, with kindness and love. Many times, our dear friends see attributes and strengths in us that we don't even see in ourselves.

Tip #2: Gratitude

If you have a hard time with self-love—and many of us do—try starting with gratitude. Being grateful for even the simplest of things has been proven to have positive benefits for health and well-being.

Remembering those good times in your life when you had a happy or soul-fulfilling experience is a great way to take care of yourself. Sit still for a few minutes and recall a happy memory, putting yourself mentally in that time and place and remembering how wonderful it felt.

I like to go to a vacation spot in my head, feel the warmth of the sunshine on my arms and face, hear the ocean waves splashing up the shore and dragging back out all the tiny shells, the birds calling, the relaxation I feel sitting in the low beach chair, under the umbrella, my mind free and clear of worry, a cold beverage in my hand. This is a good memory, and going there in my mind is de-stressing, a powerful form of self-care. What is a happy memory for you?

When we put energy towards things we're grateful for, we attract more things with that same energy to our lives.

Tip #3: Start moving

When feeling blue or depressed, do not stay in bed. Even the act of getting up, taking a shower, and getting dressed will help your overall mood. Even if it doesn't feel like it, mild activity gets the blood flowing in your body and brain.

So, leave the house every day. Go to work, it is a positive for you. If you work from home, run an errand, walk outside, go see your friend or mother, get out of the house daily. It does you no good when you are feeling down to succumb to doing nothing. It will not help you feel better, or live better.

My hope is that you feel the need to move each day, and get out walking, biking, swimming, or going to the gym at least three times a week. Getting your blood pumping through your brain and body is self-care. Carving out that time in your week is not selfish—it is necessary to live well and be well.

Tip #4: Creating a positive mindset – affirmations

When you love yourself, it is easier to hold supportive beliefs and thoughts about your life, your emotions, and your aging body.

In ancient folklore, there are three stages to a woman's life—Maiden, Mother, and Crone. The young girl, the woman in the reproductive zone, and the old woman.

Reject the negative ideas and concept of the old Crone while embracing the positive. The Crone is often depicted as disagreeable or obstructionist, but in some traditions, the Crone means wisdom, freedom, and personifying the positives of aging. Just because my body does not look like it did in my 20s does not mean I am worthless, ugly, fat, and put out to pasture. No! If you find yourself telling yourself these types of negatives, pull it back, and knock it off.

Yes, your body is changing, but step into that power you have as a woman who is evolving and growing. It is only negative if you say and believe it is so—so silence that negative voice, and replace it with words of positive affirmation.

Do I mourn that tight, smaller, perkier body? Yes, for a moment, and then I'm done! I'm moving on. I'm honoring all the things about myself that I did not know when I was younger. Look at your life, the relationships you've had, the experiences you've been through. In self-reflection, you can see how you have learned from them, and that wisdom is something to love.

Affirmations are simply short sentences or phrases to be read aloud that help your mind focus on how you want to feel. Post these positive thoughts at your workspace, or somewhere you will see them every day. Say them out loud—when we tell ourselves something in our own voice, it resonates the most deeply! Commit to saying a phrase or two out loud to yourself while looking in the mirror each morning, as part of your self-love practice.

Here are some examples to get you started:

I am enough just as I am

I am magnificent

Loving myself helps me fully love others

Today I will love myself

My body and brain are working hard for me

Taking care of me is loving me

Don't you feel a bit better just reading through these statements? Use these affirmations, or write a few of your own, and feel your attitude towards yourself improve.

Tip #5: Support

Part of self-care is surrounding yourself with people who support you. Consciously do an assessment of the people you hang with the most. Do they support you, or bring you down?

Recognize the folks in your life who seem to always have negative things to say, negative attitudes about you, your actions, or life in general—you know, the ones who are always taking energy and joy from you. The ones you know are not on your "team." Don't hang with them. Instead you need those people in your circles of friends, colleagues, Facebook community—anywhere you connect with people—who have your back.

Support can also mean finding other professionals to help you out. Perhaps finding a good therapist to be able to sort things through with, or hiring a house cleaner twice a month to support you in having more time to care for yourself, or reaching out to an acquaintance who has gone through what you may be going through and asking for their story and advice. Create that circle of folks who help you and support the unique, incredible woman that you are.

There are many ways to find your tribe and begin to gather supportive people around you. Join a group to learn something. What interests you? Learning to belly dance? Raising llamas? Making quilts? Taking a class at your local college? Building furniture? The list is endless, and the thing that matters is you finding like-minded people to hang with and who have positive supportive energy.

Online groups and forums are also powerful ways to connect with supportive people. No matter where you live today, you can jump on the Internet and find groups of folks who are interested in the very things you are. Science tells us that these online groups can be beneficial to you as an individual and provide positive links to general feelings of well-being (4).

Many folks also find encouragement and comfort from connecting with friends or classmates from the past. They share your memories and know parts of your history that current friends and acquaintances do not. The rule of thumb is, do you feel supported by these folks, and are they on your team? If so, strengthen your bond with them.

Tip #6: Give yourself some space

Space to slow down, space to breathe, space to move at a different pace. If tasks feel too large to tackle, you can get a better handle on things by breaking the tasks down into smaller pieces. Then just do what you can, as you can. Check each task off, and perhaps reward yourself for moving forward even when you feel like you're moving through sludge!

Give yourself time. Moods don't change in a flash when you are down, but they also always do pass. You will feel better again soon, maybe even later this week. It takes time for your brain and body to shift.

If you have a major decision to make (at work, in your home life, with your significant others) postpone the decision until you feel better. If you are looking at a major transition and are not ready to make the decision, reach out to others for advice, those in your trusted circle who will see your situation with a more objective view.

Tip #7: Medical/professional care
Oral contraceptives or antidepressants?

For some women, a low dose OC helps regulate hormones enough to stabilize moods. There have been in recent years, and still are, major controversies over this treatment. You have to decide with your medical provider if the benefits of taking estrogens outweigh the risks. To be sure, prescriptive OCs have undergone major changes since the "horse urine" scandal of the 1990s. The hormone therapies today are derived from chemical or plant-based substances. Ask about this.

Here is a direct quote from the North American Menopause Society, the bible of all things menopausal:

For perimenopausal mood swings, some experts recommend a low-dose oral contraceptive (OC)—even if contraception is not desired. These estrogen-progestin pills provide continuously stable hormone levels and may control mood swings. Plus, they provide other health benefits such as regulation of uterine bleeding and decreased risk for uterine and ovarian cancer. Smokers over age 35 should not use OCs (5).

According to the Journal of the American Medical Society, it may be beneficial for some women who are suffering from menopausal blues and mild to moderate depression to take an antidepressant. Be sure to check with your medical provider to see if this might be a supportive option for you (6).

Sometimes we need this kind of pharmaceutical help to get us through a season of menopausal transition. Exploring options that work for you is an important part of loving yourself and being your own advocate.

Traditional or alternative medical providers

When seeking a traditional or alternative medical provider, it is important to find a provider that understands the intricacies of hormonal balance and the unique changes happening in a woman's body during this stage of life. All are not the same, nor do they all share similar mindsets or knowledge about what a woman goes through during this transitional time. I suggest you do some searching and look for medical providers who are knowledgeable and sympathetic to the real changes women go through. Some options might be:

Integrative medicine providers

Chinese or Eastern medicine providers

Naturopathic Physicians

Herbal Medicine specialists

Women's Health specialists

Acupuncturists

Massage Therapists

Counselors

During my journey, I sought out and received advice and treatment from non-traditional medicine providers, because my traditional doctor and clinic couldn't provide me with strategies that worked.

I have benefitted from acupuncture, a Nurse Practitioner who specializes in women's health, and massage therapists.

Seeing a counselor or psychologist may also be helpful if you experience the Basement Blues consistently or episodically. A good therapist can help us see things clearly, or differently, relieving stress and anxiety.

If you already have a medical provider who is tuned in and gets you—fabulous! But if you need to find someone else to help you figure it all out, I encourage you to take this step in self-care and find a practitioner who will work with you to find solutions specifically for you.

Google women's health specialists in your area, ask your friends and colleagues for good referrals, and use the North American Menopause Society's "Find a Menopause Practitioner" search engine to give you ideas of where and with whom to start in your area (7).

The Fantastic Four play very important roles in lifting this symptom of sadness. You'll want to ensure that your body is receiving the nutrients it needs to maintain a positive mental state—Omega 3s, Vitamin D, and whole, fresh produce are vital to getting you back to your happy self—along with adequate sleep and exercise. Make sure to check out the appendix for these valuable resources.

Let's check back in with Elaine for an example of how she used some of these strategies to overcome the Basement Blues.

Elaine had been involved in theater during college, but it had been years, decades since she'd done anything theatrical. She decided that to try supporting her mental health and lifting herself out of the

Basement Blues, she would take a shot at something new, something that had always interested her. She took a risk and auditioned for a local theater show. She was cast! Since then, she has become a house-on-fire for the theater. Her blues have lifted. With the return of Elaine's easy, happy demeanor, she has made all kinds of new friends, working alongside of them, learning lines, music, and dance moves together—she has created a new community of Team Elaine. This is part of her self-care: doing things she loves, that make her happy, and surrounding herself with others who truly love her. Way to go Elaine!

Where is your posse? Your tribe? The ones who have your back? Find them, nurture those relationships, and love yourself by spending time with them. You will soon be out of the Basement Blues too.

Take Action

- **Get moving.** Get up out of bed. Get up from the chair. Engage in mild to moderate exercise. Walk until you feel ready for more. When feeling blue, you've got to move.
- **Pick out three positive affirmations for yourself and write them down.** Put them where you see them every day. At least once a day, say them out loud.
- **Hang out with someone who really likes you and sees your value.** Ask them what they like about you. Smile. Believe them.
- **Be a detective.** Search out providers who support you and get you.

For you and Elaine and the multitude of women suffering with these symptoms of perimenopause, you can bust out of the Basement Blues. Incorporate some of these daily practices now; take time for positive affirmations, cultivate supportive relationships, and bring feel-good activities into your day. If you have these healthy habits as a foundation, you'll have the positive practices already in place for when you are taken hormone hostage by the blues. You got this!

UH OH...

Chapter Four

Periods Unleashed

Meet Helen

Helen is no damsel in distress; she is one of the highest paid consultants in Boston, and she got there by working hard and playing hard. Helen is 52 years old and a proud, confident, highly sexual woman. A self-proclaimed "try-sexual" (meaning she'll try anything at least once), Helen puts the "casual" in casual sex and often catches herself grinning, thinking of the fun she has just had with one suitor or another. Life is good for Helen.

Lately however, Helen has been experiencing frustrating, fluctuating periods, a clear sign of perimenopause.

Story

I consider myself a woman who can deal with most anything. For example, my job. It demands a lot from me. I travel often, taking my clients out to the best restaurants, all while looking my best. I've pretty much got it dialed in; I know what to pack, which shoes to go with which outfit, which airlines will be most likely to bump me up to first-class, and how to shuffle time zones. See? Dialed.

But seriously, what is with my periods?

I flashback to a recent flight to London. The seatbelt sign had just turned off and I was looking forward to a cocktail and couple of chick flicks. Suddenly, I sneezed, and as I did, I felt a gush that could only mean: my period. F*@K! What was happening? Until recently, my body has always been predictable. My periods come every 28 days, like clockwork. This happened to be only a week after my last period and I had no idea what the EFF was happening with me.

I coyly made my way to the airplane lavatory to deal with myself. As I sat on the toilet, I thought of my body and my periods, and my mind began to wander to the day of that very first one...

I started menstruating at 12 years old, specifically on the last day of my seventh-grade year. I'll never forget it because it was our annual "Field Day." Field day was my favorite day. It was filled with three-legged races and all kinds of fun stuff. I was so excited because my 12-year-old self was a leggy, freckle-faced kid and I could run like the wind!

I woke up that Field Day morning discovering a red, rusty, tennis-ball sized spot on my sheets. I was confused and worried. How was I going to wear my cute outfit, run, and be free? Biting my bottom lip to keep from crying, I went to find my mother.

My mom smiled warmly and hugged me. She talked about how normal it was and how I was becoming a woman. A WOMAN? No. I wanted none of this. She handed me a Cadillac-sized pad and a sanitary belt. Geez, does anyone even remember those awful things? I remember them to be medieval torture devices that always made me feel dirty and gross. I wonder if they even make those anymore? Probably not, because of a little invention called adhesive, which now lines the underside of such pads.

Anyway, with my elastic belt around my waist, a humongous pad threaded onto it with girdle-like fasteners, it felt as if I had a fluffy couch between my legs. I stood in front of the full-length mirror and burst into tears. How was I going to run with a couch between my legs?!

There was no three-legged race for me that year—but there was an afternoon of hot tea and permission to lie on the couch and read comic books. I guess it wasn't ALL bad.

Back to the airplane toilet: I thought about how meaningful it is to have my period story. I wondered if all women remember theirs like I do.

Look. Whatever. I need my periods to be predictable. It's hard enough keeping and maintaining power in my work world, inhabited mainly by men. Every day I walk the line of having to be a charming hard ass. The last thing I need is an unexpected visit from "Aunt Flo." I never know when I am going to start my period anymore. It just shows up with no warning. None of the usual pre-menstrual bloating or irritability, which are the things that used to clue me in that my period was coming.

My period now laughs in the face of any schedule. This year alone I have bloodied bedsheets in Buenos Aires, Las Vegas, and Cleveland. I've taken to traveling with an extra pair of panties and baby wipes, because I never know when I'll need a quick clean-up. The worst part is that I don't feel very sexy when my period just shows up unannounced. Sex is important to me. I love it. This sudden change is messing with my confidence and my sex life.

Each time my period sneaks up on me, I am that 12-year-old girl all over again, wanting to cry and escape into comic books. I've got to figure out how to get my groove back, and fast.

Sip

Hormone Happy Hour

We hear you Helen. These kinds of sneaky surprises can catch us all off guard. No matter what's happening with your periods, whether you are experiencing some, none, volcanic eruptions, or a trickling creek, it's time to relax and take the stress off. These recipes were chosen mainly for their vibrant color, giving us a positive to focus on with the red-orange glow. Get ready to shake-it-up and let the good times flow.

Blood Orange Martini

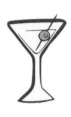

2½ oz citrus vodka
2 oz orange juice
2 oz cranberry juice
Grenadine
Splash of lemon lime soda
Blood orange or tangerine

Shake everything but soda together with ice and pour into a frosted glass. Top with soda. Garnish with a wheel slice of blood orange or tangerine.

Blood Orange Mocktini

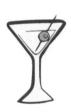

2½ oz lemon lime soda
2 oz orange juice
2 oz cranberry juice
Grenadine
Blood orange or tangerine

Shake juices and grenadine together with ice. Stir in soda and pour into a frosted glass.

Shake, stir, sip, sigh, enjoy. This period of janky periods won't last forever, and you've got the strategies to get through it.

Science of Why

You are entering the era of life called Freedom! Freedom from periods, freedom from the worry of getting pregnant when you don't want to. Freedom from buying pads, and tampons, and all the necessities of taking care of blood coming from your vagina. It's all good! Getting there can be a bit surprising, and rocky, but the journey is worth it.

Health Class

Your reproductive system is shutting down. It generally takes two to ten years before we reach the no-flow zone. Remember when you first started learning about why we get periods in the first place? Maybe it was in a health class at school, or your sister, or friend, or in an awkward discussion with your mom. Hopefully, you got some of the science from somewhere. Here's what happens: the body gets to puberty and starts releasing eggs from the ovaries (approximately one a month, usually alternating from the left to right ovary). The egg travels down the fallopian tube and free falls into the uterus. Every month, the body then builds up this nice, cushy lining, like a fuzzy comforter all around the inside of the uterus, in case the egg gets fertilized by sperm. Because if fertilization happens, the egg, now called a zygote—the egg and sperm together—then buries itself into that nice cozy lining, and thus starts the process of creating. Meanwhile, all those months the egg is not fertilized, the body flushes out the uterine lining, as well as the egg, through your vagina—and you get your period (1). Hello again!

This is all done and regulated by hormone levels. The estrogens regulate ovulation, or the shutting down thereof, and progesterone is in charge of laying down the layers in the uterus, and then getting rid of the layers, i.e. menstruation. When hormone levels are shifting, many women experience changes in the patterns and/or flow of their periods. When estrogens shift, your body will release eggs accordingly, sometimes closer together, which causes you to have a period more than once a month, and sometimes much farther apart. As a woman gets closer to true menopause (no periods for twelve months), the menstruation becomes farther and farther apart, until the day you are done with it all. Progesterone tries to balance the estrogens, but often they are out-of-balance and you enter into a phase of "estrogen dominance," which can also affect the timing of the period flow (2). Heavier or lighter flows, shorter or longer periods of time in between periods. This can be most annoying and embarrassing!

One June, during my own march towards freedom, I was at a champagne reception for a national board I served on. I showed up in a cute white skirt and bright orange jacket combo. As I was sipping champagne and chatting up a major sponsor, I felt the telltale squirt of my vagina depositing something wet and not entirely liquid into my panties. Uh, OH. I had not had a period for 15 months and thought I was so done and already in the freedom zone. Nope! White skirt, red period, no supplies of any kind. I had to discreetly excuse myself and go around to other female board members asking if they had anything I could use. After the fourth person said no, they had nothing on them, and as more gunk was flowing out, I finally found a friend with an extra tampon. Thank god! I rushed into the restroom, and took care of it the best I could—you know the drill: the wiping of yourself and the panties, the wadding up of the tissue paper to soak up the wet, trying to decide if you should ditch the panties altogether and go Commando the rest of the day (or would that make it more likely that a stain would soak through the white skirt?), the scheming of when you can next get to a private place to change your panties and wash-up properly.

I made it through that episode, but had many other surprise periods during my journey before I was finally through and truly free. The medical definition of menopause is no period for twelve months and you are done with it, so why did I bleed again at 15 months? Good question. Hormone balance is not an exact science, and for some reason my body decided it was not quite done; some hormone cocktail inside of me orchestrated another period. Lovely.

Transition

In the earlier years of transition, you see more changes, particularly with the speeding up of time in between periods, so they come more often. They become erratic in timing, so predicting when you will "start" becomes near impossible. During later transition, times in between periods generally become longer and longer. This can be stressful, as it is still possible to conceive during this transitional phase. Birth control methods must be employed if you are having sex, as you are still at risk of getting pregnant. When you have a period, that means there was an egg released, but the older we get the older our eggs get. Did you know a baby girl is born with all the eggs she will ever have already inside her ovaries? Amazing. While men make new sperm every day? Yes, it's true—but that's another story... The point is, your eggs get old. They are as old as you are, and in general, older eggs do not make for healthy pregnancies and pregnancy outcomes. Thus, the ticking clock syndrome is what many women who want to get pregnant in their mid-to-late thirties feel.

So, what did I do the first time my period didn't come for 60 days? Right! I got a pregnancy test immediately!

Remember, it is the estrogen levels that prompt the start of a period cycle, and as we get older, our periods decrease as the estrogen levels in our bodies gradually decline.

Strategy

Tips for Living Your Best Self
Tip #1: Always be prepared

Truth is, you never know when the flow or spurt or gush will happen. I recommend always carrying an essential emergency pack: tampon case, wet wipes, clean panties, Motrin, and chocolate—because after an embarrassing event like that, you need some comfort!

Tip # 2: Keep track

According to the North American Menopause Society, a perimenopause diagnosis is made through your age, menstrual history and self- reporting (3). In order to self-report, we must keep track of what our bodies are doing, including how we feel emotionally and physically, the dates when we menstruate, and what our periods are like. These pieces of information are useful in getting a diagnosis of perimenopause(4). When you know what's going on, you are more empowered to deal with it!

Keep a calendar—paper or electronic, whatever floats your boat— and keep track of days you bleed, whether it was heavy or light, bright red or brown. Also keep track of your symptoms like cramps and that drag-down-moving-through-mud-tiredness that sometimes comes on. It is helpful to track your feelings too, as it contributes to your self-empowerment to know what is happening in your own body. This awareness can help you warn or explain what is going on with you to your loved ones, both emotionally and physically.

Tip #3: Birth control

I know, I know, we are leaving the reproductive zone, transitioning to a life free of periods, so why would a woman use oral contraceptives during this phase of life?

The argument can be made for three reasons:

1) Period regulation. The use of oral contraceptives (OC) during the transitional years can be helpful when dealing with irregular, gushing periods. The hormones within the OC serve to regulate periods in this stage of life, similar to how they regulate periods during the reproductive phase of a women's life.

2) You can still get pregnant during perimenopause. So, you have to do something to protect against an unwanted pregnancy if you are still enjoying sex (and I hope you are), and some women choose to use oral contraceptives for this purpose. In fact, the Mayo Clinic recommends oral contraceptives until the age of 55 as being a positive and normal choice for many women (5).

3) OC can help regulate those irritating hot flashes and night sweats. For some women, going the traditional OC route through perimenopause is welcomed, as it can help with more than just period regulation. This is a decision you must make in consultation with your health care provider, as long-term use of OC also has its negative effects.

Conversely, there are many different herbs and plants that can moderate or help lessen your periods. I recommend consulting a naturopath or herbalist provider to see if this might be a good option. I do know women who have had their periods stopped completely, putting them directly into the postmenopausal zone, by using certain natural remedies. My mom is one. She was at the end of menopause transition with severe, heavy, non-stop bleeding. She went to an herbalist, and whatever he gave her, it stopped her bleeding completely. Unfortunately, that specific herbal recipe has been lost with time, or I would tell it here. The point being, alternative remedies may be helpful to you.

This argument for or against OC, and when to stop using it if you already are, is waged between traditional western medicine and alternative therapy methods. The decision also has to do with your own predisposition—are you more inclined towards traditional methods in healthcare, or do you prefer more natural, herbal, and alternative methods?

The Fantastic Four play a role here as well. Keep exercising and get that heart pumping, even as blood is pumping out of you. It can reduce the unpleasant symptoms of bloating, cramping, and irritability. Give your body the nutrients it needs by eating optimally, try to get the sleep your body craves, and possibly look at hormone replacement therapy. These all can be positive players as your body works to shut down the reproductive zone and stop the periods altogether.

Take Action

- **If you are still having periods, start keeping track.** Write down the day you start, how long you have a flow, what the flow is like. Heavier or lighter? What color is it, more red or brown-rust? Is it thicker or thinner?
- **Put together your own menstrual emergency kit so you will always be prepared for the unexpected.** You may even be able to help a fellow traveler out.
- **Discuss with your medical provider what would be the best option for you regarding birth control during this transitional phase.**

Bleeding all over and at unexpected times is super annoying, especially in social situations. But irregular periods are a hallmark sign of going through perimenopause as your body is doing its work of shutting down the reproductive zone. That is something to be celebrated! So, be prepared, keep track, and empower yourself with knowledge about your own body to beat this Hormone Groan.

Chapter Five

The Hot Flash

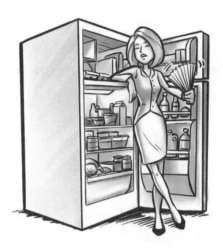

Meet Jennifer

Jennifer is smart, efficient, and the type of woman who is annoyed by anything that slows down her progress. There are few things that frustrate Jennifer more than a slow-moving line or a traffic jam. It's important for her to stay on top of remembering things. This includes your birthday and my anniversary. She is an over-achiever, and works hard at getting it ALL done. Feeling out of control is especially challenging for Jennifer, so you can imagine how hard it was for her when she began to experience symptoms of perimenopause, particularly hot flashes.

Story

My name is Jennifer, and I am 48 years old (dabs head with a tissue). I have always prided myself on being well-organized and capable, but lately, it's been hard to keep up with my life.

Currently, I am the reluctant leader of my city's planning commission. My lack of enthusiasm for this job comes from the fact that I am a true introvert. I simply don't enjoy being in front of people. In fact, getting up in front of a crowd makes me so nervous that I can actually hear the beating of my own heart—I'm just sure it's going to pop right out of my chest!

Jeez (fans self with papers), is it warm in here to you?

Anyway, when I'm presenting to an audience, my legs start shaking and my voice retreats somewhere into the recesses of my throat. My speaking gets squeaky, and I stutter as I try to talk to my audience. I've been so nervous (dabs head with a tissue again) that I have literally finished a presentation and found that I can't remember what I just said. For these reasons, even though my coworkers tell me I am the natural choice to be the chair, I don't think I'm the best choice for this position.

What else? Oh, I have always been 20 to 40 pounds overweight, as determined by any height-weight-body mass index-calculating tool you can find, and (takes off her blazer) I am constantly working to "slim down." It feels—especially lately—like it's a battle I can't win, which is hard for me to accept. I mean, the endless cycle of diets, the not–eating–certain–foods, the eating–only–certain–foods–at-certain–times, the fasting, the counting, the shakes and supplements. I see myself gleefully greeting that magic number on the scale as I meet my goal, only to have it disappear again in a matter of weeks, eventually creeping back up to an even larger size. It is SO demoralizing.

Is there a place I can hang this? It really is quite warm in here.

It is really important to me to at least try and control as much as I can. For example, that blazer you're hanging up is from a designer collection that I just adore. I am meticulous in what I can control about my appearance. From the correct fit of my clothes to my matching shades of lipstick and nail polish, I consider myself the consummate professional.

I wonder if the heat is up too high (fans self with clipboard). Would you mind checking?

Where was I? Oh, yes. My control issues. I find that I can usually pull myself together—but lately, THIS happens (points to the obviously wet spots soaking her shirt). I guess they are called hot flashes. For me, I know they're coming because I feel a warm flush starting up my body and within 60 seconds I am just dripping with sweat!

Not only am I often a sweaty mess, but my face will suddenly, and for no reason, turn 12 shades of crimson red. I try to camouflage the redness with layers of foundation and powder, but the sweat somehow seeps through any efforts I make. I often end up wiping it all off. Sometimes, if I'm lucky, it isn't so extreme and I can get away with blotting myself with a tissue or take comfort from a nearby fan, but when a bad one happens, it is painfully humiliating. Just yesterday, I felt the flush of a hot flash as I tried to conduct a meeting, and as I lifted my arm to make a point, I noticed (only after everyone else did), that there was literally a pool of sweat on the table left behind from my arm.

(Pauses to take a long drink of water.)

These episodes are becoming more and more frequent, and other than living in front of a fan or moving to the North Pole, I'm not sure what to do.

Sip

Hormone Happy Hour

Let's get Jennifer a yummy, cooling drink as she sits down to figure out what to do about all these hot flashes, and how to navigate this Hormone Groan. These recipes utilize healing properties of cucumbers. Just as cucumber slices placed on your eyelids can reduce puffiness, (yes, they can—they are an anti-inflammatory) they also provide vitamins and minerals to help you stay healthy and cope with all these hot flashes. Bring on the vitamins C, K, B5, the potassium and magnesium. Let's cool this body down.

Cool as a Cucumber Martini

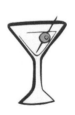

2½ oz vodka
1 oz simple syrup
½ half fresh lime, juiced
2 slices peeled English cucumber
3 drops green Tabasco
Fresh cilantro

Muddle cilantro, cucumber, lime juice, and syrup. Add vodka. Stir and strain. Add Tabasco. Garnish with a cucumber wheel and sprig of fresh cilantro.

Cool as a Cucumber Mocktini

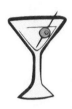

3 oz soda water
3 oz lemonade
¾ oz fresh lime juice
3 slices peeled English Cucumber
3 drops green Tabasco
Fresh Cilantro

Muddle cilantro, cucumber, lime juice, and syrup. Add lemonade and soda water. Stir and strain. Add Tabasco. Garnish with a cucumber wheel and sprig of fresh cilantro.

Or you can make cucumber water by smashing and essentially pureeing a cucumber through something called a chinois, which is a fancy word for a sieve—you know, those cone-shaped ones that have tightly woven mesh on them. Just peel and cut up the cucumber into small chunks and mash it around in there. The resulting cucumber water can then be used to mix up your Cool as a Cucumber Martini or Mocktini.

WARNING: the exertion needed to chinois your cucumber will most likely cause you to hot flash!!

Ahhh... Better already. Let's get some learning on.

Science of Why

Jennifer needs some relief. Let's find out why we do get hot flashes, and what we can do to cool the body down.

The medical description of hot flashes are recurrent, transient episodes of flushing, and a sensation of warm to intense heat on the upper body and face often followed by chills. No kidding?! I know many of you can relate to Jennifer, with the incredible heat and the aftereffects of a hot flash soaking your clothes, undergarments, and skin.

Your Body's Furnace

The temperature center of your body is a gland within your brain called the Hypothalamus. Much like the furnace in your home, the hypothalamus is responsible for regulating your body's temperature. We have learned with some of the other menopausal symptoms that the brain is extremely sensitive to hormonal changes, affecting the neurotransmitters and many other brain and bodily systems. While the science is not exact, most believe that as a woman's estrogen levels fall, the hypothalamus detects too much body heat, sending a cascade of communications to raise your heart rate and dilate your blood vessels to get more blood flowing through the body, which helps dissipate or get rid of the excess heat. This then allows for the body's natural cooling system to be activated—sweat. The goal of the hypothalamus is to get the body temperature back to a normal state, and this goal causes the sweaty, sticky, uncomfortable hot flashes [1,2].

We hosted a graduation party for our daughter when she finished her degree at the university. We had everyone over, our friends, her friends, her Dad's whole family, grandparents—you get the picture. Lots of people, many who don't normally hang out together (a stress inducer in and of itself). On this, the hottest day of that year, our furnace broke, which means we had no AC, which means the inside of our house was as hot as outside. It was 103 degrees Fahrenheit. There was no relief, and everyone, not just me and my menopausal friends, were dripping in sweat. Much like your home's furnace, your brain acts as your body's furnace, and when it is not working optimally, here come the hot flashes and night sweats, increasing in severity and frequency like tsunami waves crashing on the beach.

The truth is, at least 75% of perimenopausal women in the United States have hot flashes, and it is the number ONE reported menopausal symptom. This intense perspiration can increase your body temperature 1-7 degrees hotter, for the brief seconds your body's heat peaks (3).

So, let's do the math: if a normal body temperature is 98.6 degrees, and it's possible you could increase your temperature by 7 degrees, that would mean that for an instant or two, your temperature could reach 105.6 degrees. HOT!!

Fortunately, we only stay at these elevated temperatures for mere moments, otherwise our brains would fry. You can see why the body goes into full put-out the-fire mode, with your own personal firefighter defense coming to town and causing you to sweat buckets in order to bring the temperature down to normal levels. I prefer to think of my personal firefighters as hunky, gorgeous, sexy men, coming to work just for my pleasure (wink). Makes the hot flash a little more bearable.

Then, naturally, the hot flash is usually followed by being chilled, as your wet skin is exposed to the air. Perfectly natural bodily response. But-oh-so uncomfortable to now be going about your day with wet bra and panties.

Another thing that happens during the hot flash is your heart rate speeds up. The speed-up range is usually 7-15 more beats per minute than your average heart rate. So, the heart races and the blood vessels dilate and you are internally screaming... and it's not from some incredible sexual encounter with your fireman.

A curious fact: while the hypothalamus regulates the body's temperature, and falling estrogen is thought to cause the hot flash, the reverse is true also; if you have too much estrogen, you are susceptible to more hot flashes. And body fat not only stores estrogens, but it can convert another hormone, DHEA (4), into more estrogen. So, more body fat = more estrogen = more hot flashes. Ha! More good news for the menopausal woman who already sees the fat stores increasing.

Strategy

Tips for Living Your Best Self

Send in the firefighters... For hot flash help, we turn to the cornerstone of the Fantastic Four, which is so important in body temperature regulation that she gets another huge shout-out here—The Queen of all hot flash helpers: EXERCISE!

Tip #1: The Queen - EXERCISE!

What? Why would exercise, which actually raises your heart rate and makes you hotter, be good for hot flashes? Let's take a closer look.

It's back to the brain and your temperature regulator, the hypothalamus. Studies show that when women engage in the types of exercise that increase their cardiovascular health, like vigorous walking, running, swimming, cycling, etc. your core temperature is increased and the circulation through your blood vessels near the skin and in your brain are enhanced, which leads the brain to have better temperature regulation (5). So, exercise is to the hypothalamus like changing the filter is to our home's furnace—it helps it run and control temperature better. Good stuff! As we have seen with so many menopausal symptoms, exercise does nothing but help us.

Simply put, we know that wacky hormone levels lead to more hot flashes—exercise helps counter the consequences of changing hormone levels, and may even increase the right type of estrogen levels, which leads to less hot flashing (6,7).

Just like any new activity, making a commitment to yourself and taking baby steps will help. In my blogs and talks, I challenge women to just 30 minutes of activity, three times a week. Exercise can be as simple as lacing up your sneakers and walking during your work breaks. I know some women who go up and down flights of stairs on their lunch hour and get a great work out, where the endorphins are flowing and the stress is relieved.

Or find a work out buddy. Just knowing someone is waiting for you to show up helps you show up and be committed. Some of my favorite exercise is walking the park near my home with a girlfriend. Not only do I get exercise, but the friendship, input, and counseling I get from walking and talking is life-affirming. Commit to getting your sexy sweat on.

Tip #2: Phytoestrogens

Phytoestrogens are substances derived from plants that act as an estrogen-like substance in the body. A whopping 40-50% of women from western countries use these and other complementary and/or natural alternatives to find relief from menopausal symptoms (8). I am one of them. Research is unclear about whether they act like bio-identical hormones with the lock and key effect at estrogen receptors, or if they work to inhibit or modulate this action, that is, stop, slow-down, or control this action (9).

There is a conflict about these substances that mainly revolves around the fact that they cannot be vetted or regulated through the FDA. This is because they are plant-based, not made from refined chemicals, so proving they will do what they claim to do, or how helpful or harmful they are, is challenging. Also, there is no consistency in the research regarding the amount or dose you should take of these substances. That's the down side. (You can read more about this in the Fantastic Four section.)

The up side is many women find relief, at least temporarily, through the use of OTC phytoestrogen supplements and, even better yet, by eating foods high in them. Women looking for natural alternatives to HRT (hormone replacement therapy) often turn to foods and herbs which contain phytoestrogens to calm menopausal symptoms, including, you guessed it, hot flash severity.

The most common places to find phytoestrogens in food are:

- fermented soy products
- whole grains
- nuts, especially walnuts
- seeds, particularly flax

You may have also heard of them in herbs and plants such as black cohosh, Dong Quai, red clover, or wild American ginseng, as well as many others. I recommend talking to a subject matter specialist at your local or online supplement store for more information on the benefits of these foods and herbs.

Many of the OTC menopausal aids, or those you hear being advertised on the radio or in your magazines, have some combination of phytoestrogens and vitamins. The effect of these phytoestrogens on YOUR body is contingent on things unique to you, like your metabolism, how your body effectively absorbs them, and your schedule for taking them.

A Word About Soy

Although soy is considered a phytoestrogen, some caution needs to be applied. Soy contains isoflavones, which are estrogen-mimicking molecules. This seems good, except non-fermented soy products can give you too many estrogen mimicking molecules, which can lead to an increased risk of estrogen-sensitive cancers like breast and uterine.

The safest way to ingest soy is by eating soy that has been fermented at least three months. Products like miso, tamari, tempeh, and tofu are considered safe soy.

In America, most soy is processed to separate the oil and the protein, but this fails to remove the toxins and anti-nutrients. In fact, the processing can leave carcinogenic residues in the product. In addition, soy that is not fermented inhibits calcium, iron, and zinc absorption in the body.

It is reported that women who eat a typical Asian diet high in fermented soy, like tofu and tempeh, have nearly non-existent hot flashes. So, the word about soy is consume it, but only the fermented varieties.

Tip #3: Clothing

It almost goes without saying that dressing in layers is the way to go during the Hot Flash Zone! It is best to wear clothing that can breathe and wick away sweat. Avoid synthetic fabrics that trap sweat, odor, and moisture. You know how uncomfortable that can be during the day—when you flash with sweat, then cool down and your undergarments and sometimes outer garments are wet. Yuck! Look for fabrics that are breathable or wicking. Many of the fabrics used today for athletic wear are good examples. Start with your base layer of underthings that are moisture wicking, so they pull the wet away from you. Layer on lightweight blouses or tops, and jackets or sweaters over that. In a professional setting, just make sure your base layer provides appropriate coverage for when you feel like "taking it all off."

Beware of 100% cotton. While it can seem a comforting and light fabric, it is "water-loving" and will trap the wet and sweat. We've all seen cotton shirts on men and women with the large, dark, wet staining—it may be OK at the gym, but we don't need our clothes screaming to the world that we are flashing. Plus, wet cotton tends to bag and bunch. Cotton synthetic blends, however, can work nicely.

And while compression panties, t-shirts, slips, and bras can help pull us in and make us feel a bit sleeker, beware those types of products that will trap the heat and sweat on your body.

Fortunately for us, there is an entire industry growing to help women who hot flash. Here are some websites to get you started, and happy shopping!

- www.cool-jams.com
- www.lusome.com/us
- hotcoolwear.com/index.php?route=product/
    product&path=59_66&product_id=85
- www.lanjetee.com
- www.knockoutpanties.com/collection.php?show=c5

Take Action

- **Make a plan for exercise.** Find a friend. Write it down. Do it.
- **Pick one or two foods high in phytoestrogens and try eating and/or cooking with them for a week or two.**
- **Go shopping for something new you can wear that will wick sweat away and make you feel good!**

Use these tips, along with all the ones listed in the chapter on Night Sweats, (as the science and mechanisms of action are basically the same) to manage the flashes and beat this hormone zone.

Chapter Six

Night Sweats

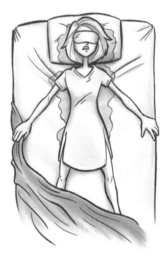

Meet Nadine

This time last year, Nadine was shopping for a wedding dress. Falling in love at this point in her life was not what she had expected, but after meeting Tim she felt younger and happier than she had in years. At 46, Nadine had a suspicion that some of her best years were in front of her. The kids almost grown, a new, true love by her side, she was ready to deal with the rest of her life. Night sweats became her biggest problem. Not so bad, right?

Story

I am SO happy. This is important, because even two years ago, I couldn't have said that. But today I can. I am HAPPY. I fell in love with my soulmate. His name is Tim.

(Begins to sing:) "I'm in love, I'm in love, I'm in love with a wonderful guy!"

Ha! See? I even sing now. It's ridiculous. He is everything I've ever wanted. We met through mutual friends, (thank you Brenda and Sean!) and the zing we both felt when our eyes met? It was electric. Love found us. If it weren't for the fact that I can't get through one damn night in my new, amazing life without sweating myself silly, I would call my life almost perfect.

We've spent the last few months working to blend our families. He has one son and I have three daughters. All the kids are active in sports or music, and with the younger two, every night holds something.

Most days involve meetings around the dining room table with Tim, trying to figure out who's driving which kid where, and for what event. Dinner, laundry, the dishes, all the details that make a household hum or crash, these are the things we spend our days navigating. I find myself enjoying it. Tim is easy-going and able to diffuse most of the kid and schedule challenges with his witty sense of humor and his "don't sweat the small stuff" attitude. I am a lucky one.

But oy, the sweats. One thing that really throws a big bucket of water (no pun intended) on this loving fire are these troubles in the bed department. Not sexually–that part is going just fine. My problem is that the sweats keep me from sleeping.

Disrupted sleep is playing havoc on my daily life. Though I'm happier than ever, I am also more tired than ever. I have always tried to get 7-8 hours of sleep a night, and even when the kids were young, I established firm bedtimes—for them and me. I worked to make our night time routine one where we had the best chance of getting the rest we all needed. When I don't sleep well, I feel as if I'm walking through mud.

I'm a happy, muddy mess.

Here is what a typical night looks like. The night sweats do their thing. I wake up and my thoughts start spiraling. I think of the million things I must do the next day. I think about what must happen so the kids have rides and snacks for their after-school events. I worry, "Am I being a great wife? Does Tim have what he needs from me?" I worry about my parents' health. I worry about money.

Anything can provoke the sweats. The blankets are too heavy, or my husband's toe brushes up against my leg. I react by waking up drenched and hotter than hell. Sweat soaks my body, the sheets, and often, poor Tim. I wouldn't mind the heat and the sweat if this was a passionate sexual encounter. But there is nothing sexy about this. I imagine, because of my age, it is a symptom of my perimenopause.

After a night sweat has wreaked its havoc, it's impossible to get comfortable. The sheets are cold and wet. And pajamas? SOAKED.

All this is to say, many days I am a wreck. I know I said I am happy. And I am happy. But I'm agitated too, because I haven't had enough decent sleep. Tim is worried because of my mood swings and short attention span. My normal capacity to keep all the balls spinning just isn't the same.

Yes, there is sometimes yelling, and sometimes tears, and my poor, dear husband must pick up the slack.

I'm worried and I'm tired.

(I'm happy too. Really, I am.)

Sip

Hormone Happy Hour

Nadine needs some cooling, mind-clearing martini time. This martini recipe is made with mint—both in the alcohol and as fresh leaves. Mint has a cooling effect, as it contains menthol, a chemical that triggers the cold receptors in your skin.

The Mocktini's green tea is also considered a "cooling food" in Chinese medicine. Add the fresh mint and you are on your way to refreshment. Let's settle in with Nadine and enjoy an ice-cold drink.

Arctic Cool Martini

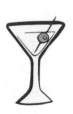
2 oz vodka

1 oz crème de menthe

2 slices fresh lemon

Fresh basil

Fresh mint

Muddle basil, mint, and two slices of lemon together. Add vodka and crème de menthe. Vigorously shake together with ice and strain. Pour into chilled martini glass. Garnish with fresh basil and mint leaves.

Arctic Cool Mocktini

4 oz soda water

4 oz green tea

2 slices fresh lemon

Honey to taste

Fresh basil

Fresh mint

Muddle basil, mint, and two slices of lemon together. Steep two mint tea bags in 8 ounces of hot water for five minutes. Discard tea bags. Add tea and a few drops of honey to muddled ingredients. Vigorously shake together with ice, strain. Pour into chilled martini glass. Top with soda. Garnish with fresh basil and mint leaves.

For a warm mocktini, leave out the soda water and shake ingredients together without ice.

Sip it, breath deep, relax, and feel your temperature chill out.

Science of Why

Remember the hypo-t thermostat in your brain from the hot flash Science of Why, when the signals in the brain activate your own personal firefighters coming to the rescue? They detect temperatures rising, like in a fire, sound the alarm, push their activity into high gear, jump into the truck, get to the scene of the fire, (increase your heart rate activity) and open the hoses to put out the flames. Once the sweat is glistening and running down every crack in your body, they roll up the hoses, close down the blood vessels, and go back to the station to await the next temperature siren.

This is the exact reason and sequence of action behind night sweats. Same thing, just that one happens while we go about our day and the other happens as we sleep.

These massive temperature fluctuations are unnecessary–don't you think? It's the imbalance of hormones tripping the hypo-t thermostat, and if we could bring more balance to the seesawing levels we could get some needed relief. We also have some control over temperature triggers that are not primarily estrogen and progesterone related.

Strategy

Tips for Living Your Best Self

Nadine, and all of us who wake up drenched at night, need some advice to live our best selves in the midst of the wet sheets and sweat-slicked skin. Keep the Fantastic Four activated and read on for some positive advice. You can also use any of these strategies to help with hot flashes, as the science is the same and cooling down is the goal.

Tip #1: Reduce stress

No kidding? Don't you feel like this piece of advice comes from everywhere? We live in such a fast-paced world with many expectations put on us as women, both externally from society and inside ourselves. The constant trying to finish the ever-growing to-do list and measuring up to some kind of ideal we mentally aspire to... Stop. Just stop. Breathe deep. Take a quiet moment for yourself, with yourself.

Stress releases neurochemicals that actually increase our core temperature and lower the temperature neutral zone, that space where you are in balance and neither sweat nor shiver. So, adopting workable strategies to reduce your stress can diminish the severity and frequency of night sweats (1). These can range from practicing meditation, to yoga, to deep breathing, to listening to music that makes you feel happy or lighthearted, to listening to a podcast that makes you laugh out loud! Anything that makes you genuinely smile or pleases your senses will relieve stress. What activities help you to relax? What gives you relief from the stressors of everyday life? These things will help reset your temperature controls to the neutral zone—the place we want to be.

Breathing can play a big role in lowering your stress levels. Research has shown that if you can "catch" a hot flash beginning to happen, taking three very deep, very long breaths can sometimes stop the flash before the sweating comes on (2). In addition, spending a few minutes each day focusing on breathing deep, inhaling for 4-5 seconds, holding the breath for a couple of seconds, and then releasing the breath slowly, has immediate results. I find myself switching to deep breathing mode when I feel the stress coming on—sitting in stop-n-go traffic, dealing with a family member who is driving me crazy, or having to practice patience when I'm rushing forward. Worth a try!

Also, it is proven that listening to music you don't like can decrease the diameter of your blood vessels and blood flow throughout the body, cascading to increased blood pressure, stress, and irritation. Hopefully, your workplace doesn't play music that irritates you all day long. Pay attention to how music makes you feel, and work to eliminate listening to the styles, songs, or artists that resonate sadness, irritation, or anger in you. One music trigger for me is my husband's musical preference for 80s rap–it sets me on edge. Hot flash city, here we come! Working to reduce stress during your waking hours will help with both hot flashes and night sweats.

Tip #2: Avoid personal triggers – physical and emotional

What did you eat or drink this evening in the few hours before bedtime? Had that third glass of wine? Decided to add raw jalapenos to the pizza at dinner? Caffeine, spicy foods, and alcohol are hot flash/night sweat triggers for many women. Pay attention to when the night sweats come, and try to remember what you ingested before bed to help understand your personal clues.

Alcohol in the evening can disrupt sleep in multiple ways, including pouring on the night sweats. Your inner thermostat is raised as your body works to metabolize it.

Spicy foods can sometimes cause a reaction in your digestive system which elevates body temperatures and may trigger flashing.

Caffeine too late in the day can mess with our sleep patterns and can also prompt the hot flash/night sweat.

Emotional stress before bed can trigger night sweats later in your sleep cycle. If you are needing to have a confrontation with a family member, or deal with a hot button topic, before bed is never a good time. If you are reading reports or listening to news that is upsetting to you, beware the night sweats later.

I have a younger brother who lives in a time zone 6 hours from me. He likes to call late in the evening, usually when I am already in bed, have already performed my sleep hygiene rituals, and have calmed myself in readiness for sleep. If I take his call, I will for sure get revved up. We are only fourteen months apart in age, and competition with each other is as ingrained as our eye color. So, he may start with something like, "I'm down to my high school weight, how're you doing?" Or talk about his latest over-the-top-super exciting adventure, asking if I've "done anything interesting lately?" I usually take the bait and off we go! He knows how to push my buttons on a variety of issues and he also knows how to make me laugh. Whether the call is positive or negative, there is no way I will fall asleep anytime soon after we talk. I made a deal with myself years ago—no late-night phone calls.

Calming your emotions before bed and setting personal boundaries is a worthwhile endeavor. Make a choice to "put away" emotionally-charged issues for the evening, and quiet your inner self. And, as I did, put the phone away and don't take calls an hour before your bed time. Even from those parents of your children's friends, or the person trying to get you to volunteer on their pet project. Who thinks calling after 9 pm is ok? It's not. Unless it is a medical emergency, the calls can wait. Read more about this in the Fantastic Four and sleep hygiene.

Tip #3: Stop smoking

An unfortunate side effect of smoking is the triggering of specific hormone changes that can cause earlier and more intense hot flashes. Just another reason to try and make this positive health choice. One woman I met recently shared her story with me. She has been having night sweats for 17 years! She is through the transition, and fully post-menopause, but still wakes up soaked at night. Unfortunately, she has smoked her entire adult life, and this most certainly is related to her flashing (3).

Tip #4: Use bamboo sheets

For the night, bamboo sheets are optimal. Bamboo fiber is naturally anti-bacterial, hypo-allergenic, and inherently resists mold, mildew, and odors. And while a bamboo stalk's exterior is tough, the inner fiber is of a porous nature. This allows bamboo fabric to have strong absorbing qualities, to be breathable, and provide excellent wicking and ventilation properties—all essential qualities of any fabric for keeping your body temperature regulated. Note: be careful of sheets that claim bamboo, but are not 100%. The blends will not be nearly as effective. Try to buy as close to 100% bamboo sheets as you can afford. They are worth it.

I use bamboo sheets and what I love the most about them is, when I wake up soaked with the night sweats, I get up to use the restroom and by the time I get back into bed, the sheets have already started to dry, so they feel just right—cool and not soaking wet. The pillowcase also has absorbed some of the sweat, so smashing my face back into it is not so bad.

Tip #5: Exercise (for more, see Tip #1 in the "Hot Flashes" chapter)

The positive effects of exercise for the menopausal woman night sweat sufferer cannot be stressed enough. Consistent, vigorous exercise helps regulate body temperature. Like keeping oil in your car engine, exercise lubes up the temperature center in your brain so it can operate more effectively. The caution here is to avoid strenuous exercise near bedtime as that can actually increase your internal temperature and possibly cause you to flash at night (4, 5). Now, a good round of sexual activity is okay before sleep, as it tends to lead to total relaxation.

Take Action

- **Practice deep, slow breathing, in and out, three times.** Breathe in to the count of 5, hold your breath for 5 seconds, slowly breathe out for 5 seconds. Do this at least 2 times daily, and as you lay down to sleep.
- **Identify your personal triggers by keeping a log for one week.** In the morning, after having night sweats, think back to the evening before—identify emotional and physical things you believe triggered the night sweats and work to eliminate those from your evening routine.
- **Go buy some bamboo sheets and pillowcases.**

We can't just make the sweats go away, but we can make some lifestyle choices that can help alleviate the frequency and/or severity of them. Most of the small changes we can make for big results work whether we are talking about night sweats or hot flashes, as they are essentially the same mechanisms causing them to happen. What works to help calm your hot flashes will also serve to help with your night sweats. We may have to give up or reduce the consumption of a few favorite things, but we also get to shop for some new items and reduce our stress. Who doesn't want that?

Chapter Seven

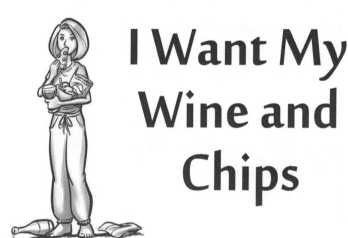

I Want My Wine and Chips

Meet Toby

Toby has spent her entire adult life focused on health and wellness. She makes her living as a documentary filmmaker and just recently received an award for her film that explores the impact of food choices on the human body. Toby is always on top of the newest health food craze and prides herself on being a positive example to family and friends. Lately, however, she finds herself having food cravings that seem to have control of her. Her newly distorted food-focus seems to be pulling her off-center. Toby is being taken hostage by her hormones. She will soon learn that her behavior around eating is not always something she can consciously regulate. Much of it is truly physiological, and as we are learning: physiology strongly impacts psychology.

Story

"Where the hell did I hide those chips?" Toby mutters distractedly to herself, heading straight through the kitchen into the pantry without even bothering to put her bag and jacket away.

"Toby, you told yourself you weren't going to do this anymore," she mutters out loud, her words and actions in complete contradiction as she scavenges through the cupboards, pushing aside boxes of high-fiber cereals and gluten free pastas in search of the holy grail: greasy potato chips.

Barbed with pangs of guilt, she finds comfort knowing that at least no one will be home for hours and she can be alone. If she doesn't have to explain it, it doesn't really count, right?

Her frenzied search causes her to knock over a bag of organic granola that opens and spills all over the pantry floor. As she reaches for the broom to sweep up the mess, she is hit with a wave of self-loathing and confusion, thinking about the healthy lifestyle she usually leads. She thinks to how often nowadays she finds herself mindlessly eating with little awareness of hunger, only to realize that the "handful" of crackers she was going to allow herself seems to turn into the entire box. "Who am I? What happened to my self-control?" At age 49, her periods were becoming irregular and her cravings were leading to compulsive junk food eating. She is binging regularly now on bread, pastries, chocolate, ice cream, and today, potato chips.

Granola swept, Toby suddenly spies the chips peeking at her from high up on the top shelf. She uses the broom handle as a tool to reach them, and she gently nudges the bag to fall into her arms. Tearing the bag open, she begins to feed herself chip after greasy, delicious chip.

It is then that she remembers the wine she bought recently. Practically dancing a jig over to the wine opener, she imagines the tastes of the salty chips combined with the sweet red wine. "NIRVAVA!!!!" she yells to no one in her empty kitchen.

Fast forward to the half-drunk bottle of red, and the empty chip bag. Toby sits on the kitchen floor and wipes the salt from her mouth with the back of her hand. She feels like she is in a constant war with her body. She thinks of all the time and energy she consumes with the maneuvering and strategizing on ways to stay away from junk food, only to lose her resolve by the day's stressful end. The cycle seems to repeat itself more and more lately. As she sips on her wine, she knows that she needs to do something different to give her body real support.

She just doesn't know how.

Sip

Hormone Happy Hour

If you can relate to Toby and the need to step away from the table, put down the bag of chips, and cork that bottle, then it's time to slow down and relax with a yummy concoction. Take away all the stress of learning—you've got more work to do to get over these cravings.

Two recipes for you this time, for both the martini and the mock-tini. One for the sweet cravers, and one for the salty cravers, so everyone can be satisfied!

Sweet Lovers:

Choc-o-love Martini

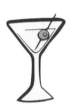

2 oz vodka

1 oz chocolate liqueur

½ oz shot Grand Marnier

Chocolate syrup

Drizzle chocolate sauce on inside of martini glass. Place all liquids in a shaker with ice. Shake vigorously. Pour into the chocolate-sauced glass.

Choc-o-love Mocktini

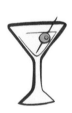

2 oz orange juice

3 oz coconut milk

Chocolate syrup

Drizzle chocolate sauce on inside of martini glass. Place all liquids in a shaker with ice. Shake vigorously. Pour into the chocolate-sauced glass.

Savory lovers:

Salted Corn Chip Martini

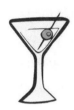

2 ½ oz vodka
1 oz dill pickle juice
1 zesty pickle spear
1 Gibson onion
1 baby corn
Crushed corn chips

Rim the glass by dipping in water and then the crushed corn chips. Shake vodka and pickle juice with ice. Pour into glass. Garnish with zesty pickle spear, Gibson onion, and baby corn a toothpick.

Salted Corn Chip Mocktini

3 oz tomato juice
1 oz dill pickle juice
1 oz Tabasco
1 zesty pickle spear
1 Gibson onion
1 baby corn
Crushed corn chips

Rim the glass by dipping in water and then the crushed corn chips. Shake tomato and pickle juices together with ice, as well as Tabasco to taste. Pour into glass. Garnish with zesty pickle spear, Gibson onion and baby corn a toothpick.

Sip, and sooth away the cravings, it's time to get some learning done.

Science of Why
Wacky Neurotransmitters

Like the mad scientist toiling over her coils of bubbling chemicals in the laboratory, your neurotransmitters have a huge role to play in the food craving game. When dopamine and serotonin (yes, you've heard of these before) get wacky, their experiments leave you wanting more—more food, more calories, more of the feeling that you need more to get full.

Let's start with a couple of definitions.

Food-Seeking Behavior

When you are cruising the kitchen cupboards for anything salty, or crunchy, or searching for that bag of holiday candy you hid, or driving past that certain fast-food place on your way home—you must have it! You will get it even when your rational mind is telling you not to. You know what this is, my pretty.

Satiety

The satisfied feeling when your belly is full after eating. You feel full. We generally like this feeling, and usually eat until we feel it.

Food-seeking behavior and satiety, in and of themselves, are perfectly normal brain-driven behaviors and signals. We need them for survival—for proper growth and repair of bone, tendons, and muscle, as well as for fueling our brain and body. It's when they are out-of-whack, or driving you to consume huge amounts of bad-for-you-food, when you don't get the message to "step away from the buffet table" in time, that they become a problem. A big problem that makes you bigger. We end up eating negative foods that are not healthy for us, and eating well beyond what we need. Bring on the bloat, weight gain, self-loathing—you know it sister!

Brain Signals

When the brain receives signals that say, "I am hungry," you want to eat. And when you are full, the brain tells you that too. That is one good reason for the age-old advice: eat slower, so the body has time to tell you you're full. Always wait 20 minutes after eating to see if you are getting the "I am full" messages, before going back for more. In fact, try to make a meal last for 20 minutes—in this fast-paced world, most meals are scarfed down in less than 10 minutes. Time it, you'll see. We eat too much and too much of the wrong things for our optimal health because, basically, the brain tells us to. Woah!

Dopamine plays many roles within the brain including influencing mood, sleep, cognition (read Brain Fog), happiness, and feelings of pleasure and reward. Pleasure and reward cycles often drive our food-seeking behavior. It is cyclical—meaning, if you have enough dopamine, the body is already feeling rewarded so there is no further need to seek out certain foods. However, if the brain is wanting a rewarding rush of dopamine, the body seeks out the greasy, salty, fat-laden, sugary substances, because as we eat these, dopamine elevates—leaving us feeling pleasure and reward. When this becomes the habit—this food-that-is-bad-for-us-or-too-much-for-us seeking behavior—the brain becomes numbed to the release of dopamine, always seeking more, so you eat even more, just like a drug addiction. At this point, you must take in more to get the feel good out of it.

This is one of the key hormones and mechanisms believed to drive the obesity rates. Scientists looked at 600 different genes to find answers to the why and how someone becomes obese. All 600 of these gene variations work on some level to impinge on dopamine release. Take home message: more dopamine means less food cravings (1).

You want high dopamine levels.

Serotonin is also closely connected to our eating habits. This hormone has been called "nature's own appetite suppressant" because if you have enough serotonin, it helps shut down the feelings that you crave more food, need more food. In other words, the appetite feels satisfied. Serotonin also helps you feel more calm, stable, energetic, and focused, which is why it is mentioned more than once regarding being a key player in other menopausal symptoms. In fact, the majority of your brain cells are influenced, either directly or indirectly, through this neurotransmitter (2).

You want high serotonin levels.

Dopamine and serotonin help control food-seeking behavior and satiety, so you want them working at full capacity for you. If they aren't, you may very well have trouble putting down the bag of chips or stepping away from the table. That's the good news here—it's not always your lack of will power—it's those wacky chemicals goofing off in the lab!

Your habits/culture around food

There's another huge why in craving certain foods: our own culture and habits around food. It's called "Classical Conditioning" and we're not talking in the weight room or at the ballet bar here. This is how you have conditioned your brain and body to want certain things, to crave them. Our emotional state has more to do with cravings than hunger (3).

The more you give in and eat what you crave, the more you will crave it. That box of saltines? How about the wine at night? Maybe you've been conditioning yourself to have one or two glasses every night—one while preparing dinner, then another while eating the meal, then cleaning up, then watching TV afterwards. Eventually, your cravings increase for it, and you want more—no, you NEED more—to get that feel-good feeling you crave, the one that used to come with the first glass! You condition your body to want and need more (4).

How many of us can start with one handful of our favorite snack, be it sweet or salty, and stop there? It takes tremendous will power.

And what are your habits around certain foods, particularly the ones that are not stellar for your health? Did you grow up soothing yourself with ice-cream or corn chips after school when you'd had a bad day? Those feelings of comfort while eating certain foods become ingrained in us, so the first step to conquering this chemical lab imbalance is to recognize your behaviors around consuming food and drink.

Strategy

Tips for Living Your Best Self
Tip #1: Change your habits (self-monitoring)

Ack!! That is sooo hard! Yes, I know. I deal with this too. As with any change you are trying to make, it helps to break it down into manageable steps as a way of helping and getting it done. The first step is you must have the "Want to." If you don't, you can put this book down right now—skip to the next chapter. If you don't have the want to, no amount of encouraging, or education, or support from others will help you change.

If you want to change your habits, here are some tips to make it a bit easier. I won't say easy—just a bit easier.

Identify the food/wine craving behavior

When do I crave it? Why do I crave it? Perhaps when you've had a hard day and you eat to reward yourself for getting through it, or when your work day is done and you want to signal your body to relax, or the house has settled down and you want to indulge in some "me time" with that bag of buttery popcorn. Identify the when, and then the why. Be honest with yourself.

Growing up, my mom made this incredible, fatty, mayonnaise-y chicken dish that I loved! It was topped with cheddar cheese and crushed up saltine crackers—my favorite. It was so good, I requested it for every birthday and special occasion. It would come out of the oven, piping hot, with all the yummy fats bubbling. Then we would dish it up over instant white rice, not brown or wild, or any other heathier, better-for-your-glycemic-control rice (we didn't even know what glycemic control was back then). Anyway, at least this casserole had broccoli in it. But it was so cooked to mush and covered with the mayonnaise and whole-can-of-cream-of-chicken-soup, you couldn't even tell it was broccoli. God, I loved that dish! So, I have seriously strong sensory memories surrounding it of good, happy times, the taste and feel in my mouth, and the crunch of the cheesy crackers. The dish is not very healthy so I don't make it much today, but the craving for it can still come over me.

Sensory memories can be a strong driver of the when, why, and what we eat. It's not just the negative, tired, or overwhelmed feelings that are tied into food—it's also the happy, feel-good memories that start a brain-chemical cascade that reinforces the craving.

What do you crave? Do you crave salt? Or fat? Or sweet? Or sour? For many people, sugar is the food they most crave, as eating it gives their brain a high and releases endorphins. You probably are well aware of your comfort foods, so go ahead and identify them now.

Make small changes to shift your habits

This can take some time, but once you recognize your habits and culture around your food choices, you can begin to modify them. When you feel a craving coming on, ask yourself, "Am I tired? Have I had enough water today?" If you can resist the urge to eat, the craving will eventually go away. Cravings are like waves of the sea; you can feel it build, and eventually it peaks, but let the water metaphorically pull away as a wave, and it will. It is helpful to distract yourself when feeling the wave crave coming: put your earphones in and listen to a happy tune, busy yourself with another activity, or turn your mind to helping someone else.

Perhaps establish an evening ritual after dinner, to reset the want for more, like brushing your teeth right away, or filling up a gigantic mug with hot water and soothing tea to sip on while you watch your favorite show, or lacing up your sneakers for a quick walk around the block. Before you realize it, the wave will have subsided and you will have conquered that craving!

Decide on Rewards

It's important to decide on rewards and treats for yourself that aren't food related. This is the fun part! What would you like? A massage? A pedicure? A long walk with a friend in the park? A new scented oil for your bath?

What will light you up as a reward? You can get creative with it: make a chart, give yourself stars on your calendar—do something visual to track your progress. You will need to put parameters on what you need to do to earn your rewards, like eating clean all week, or only having one glass of wine a night for ten days. Figure out what you want and what you think deserves you getting there. Then do it. Then reward yourself.

Tip #2: Support your brain chemistry

We want those feel-good, "help me make good choices" dopamine and serotonin firing away! Here are a few time and science tested strategies to get those chemicals bubbling in our brain:

Set goals and work toward them

Our brain is wired in such a way that, as you meet goals through-out the day, it releases more dopamine. You get a little pump of the stuff every time you check something off your list or meet one of your reward parameters we talked about before. Think of the "rush" you get when you meet a goal that has taken effort, time, strategy, and maybe some fear, like finishing a 5k, or acing an interview. When you break down your goals into smaller, achievable units, you set yourself up for success, and more dopamine!

Practice gratitude

When we reflect on what we are grateful for, our brain releases serotonin, which lifts our mood and stabilizes the brain against the cravings. It doesn't have to be an hour of meditation, but a simple daily practice, maybe when you are driving to work, or when you are drinking your morning coffee. Think of a happy memory, when you really enjoyed yourself, or something you have achieved that you are proud of. In this fast-paced world, we forget to slow down and reflect on things we have experienced, accomplished, and enjoyed. When we do reflect, we then create mental pictures of good times, people we love and who love us, and serotonin flows. A yoga instructor I once had would end her session with this phrase, which I believe helps us stay in the moment and reflect on the good in our lives:

Be grateful today for who you are, and are not.

Be grateful today for what you do, and do not.

Be grateful today for where you are, and are not.

Eat for brain health

The Fantastic Four is chock full of ideas on what to eat, and not to eat, in order to support your brain health. Turn there now for these strategies under Food Choices. In addition, Tip #4 below, which has the specifics on gut health, will support brain health as well.

Tip #3: Exercise

You know she is The Queen. Not only does vigorous exercise help elevate dopamine and serotonin, it also releases endorphins, another class of neurotransmitters that work in conjunction with dope and sero to raise the feel-good within your brain (5). The science is not exact, but studies do show that exercise increases the firing rates of serotonin, which results in more serotonin being made and released into your brain. In addition, exercise elevates tryptophan, which is a precursor to serotonin, meaning we have to have the one chemical to make the other. More tryptophan = more serotonin = more nerve endings talking with each other = better mood and control over food cravings (6). Plus, when you meet your exercise goals and enjoy how good you feel, more dopamine is released.

Tip #4: Pay attention to your gut health

Gut Health = Brain Health. The good news is, all the ways to support your GI tract during your emotional bitch rages (check out Chapter Two), are the same for your brain here in reducing cravings. Remember, the GI (or Little Brain) is full of nerve endings, and gut health is directly related to brain health. In fact, up to 90% of the feel-good chemical serotonin is made in the enteric nervous system of the gut. When your gut is producing more serotonin, it communicates with the brain to make more serotonin. This is what we want, the body and brain working in harmony and supporting one another. How do you get your gut to produce optimum levels of serotonin? It focuses back to what you are eating and not eating.

The big four are:

(1) Taking pro-biotics, either through a supplement, or active cultures like yogurt

(2) Taking an Omega 3 supplement, and/or eating more Omega 3 rich foods like salmon and walnuts

(3) Eating more fiber, preferably through 4-6 servings of fresh fruits and vegetables a day, or fiber-rich grains like oatmeal and quinoa

(4) Drinking more water, as it does amazingly good things for your gut

Water helps break down your food, releasing the nutrients into your body, and helps keep your stool soft and ready to be eliminated. The traditional quantity for water is 8 ounces, 8 times a day. A newer recommendation for water consumption is this: weigh yourself (I know, this can be painful!) and divide the amount by 2 (so if the scale says 180/2 = 90.) So, 90 ounces of water a day for you (7). Drinking enough water will also help calm your food cravings and help with weight management.

Finally, stop eating things that make your gut upset—you know what those items are. They might be some of the very foods you crave, but if they lead to gas and bloating, or constipation and diaharea you've got to cut them from your diet.

For more support with this, turn to the Fantastic Four section. Establishing positive behaviors with exercise, nutrition, and sleep will be especially helpful with food cravings.

It takes conscious effort, but I promise, the more you reinforce new habits, the easier it will become. You will still mess up, and you will still make the not-healthy choice, but you will find you are doing it less. You are getting un-stuck. You are beating the Hormone Groan of food cravings. That's something to celebrate!

Take Action

- **Do some detective work to figure out what foods you crave, when you crave them, and what you think triggers the cravings.** Write it down. You may need to keep a food diary for a week, to track what you are eating, and when, and why.

- **Decide on two strategies you can implement to reduce the likelihood of you caving into the cravings.** Will you take a walk after dinner? Will you call a friend to check in with them? Practice doing them, and get your dope on.

- **Determine your reward for meeting a food behavior goal.** Write your desired behavior change down and what you need to do to earn your reward. For example, "I will by-pass the donuts and cookies in the work lunch room every day this week." Then go after it! Another dopamine raising strategy.

- **Sweat to get your dopamine and serotonin levels up through the roof!** Put exercise in your calendar this week, aim for at least three days of 30 minutes of movement. Make dates with yourself, and keep them.

- **Spend 5 minutes a day reflecting on what you are grateful for.** Name them out loud, write them down. Soon, your serotonin will be flowing freely.

To beat the Hormone Groan with cravings, it helps to understand yourself, and recognize why and when you want these foods and sugary or alcoholic drinks. Take positive steps to support your brain and GI health, work to stop the destructive behavior, and recognize how good you feel when you have even one day of success. Celebrate that! You are beating the Hormone Groan of food cravings.

Chapter Eight

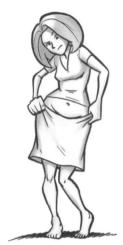

Back Fat and Jelly Rolls

Perimenopausal weight gain is very common; it's our body's way of adapting to new hormone levels as we leave our reproductive years behind.

It may be common, but it ain't easy, ladies.

What with the constant emphasis in our culture for women to be thin, and beautiful, and fit, and smart, and PERFECT, it can be especially difficult for women to experience this wholly natural, biological way our maturing bodies physically change. To represent a more diverse picture of menopausal weight gain, let's consider the experiences of three very different women, all unique in body type and activity levels, who are discovering that they need help to restore hormonal balance and deal with their growing midsections during this time of transition.

Meet Linda

42-year-old Linda is the vibrant life of any party—and we usually find that she's the one who is hosting! She knows how to bring people together and she works hard to make sure everyone has a good time. Lately, she finds it hard to maintain her "life is to be celebrated" attitude because when she looks in the mirror, she sees how her body is changing, and she doesn't like it one bit.

Story

I was never a skinny person. But lately the ten-pounds I've needed to lose has become twenty—OK—thirty pounds. Suddenly I find myself looking in the mirror wishing I could have my old body back.

Since my 40th birthday, the weight just seems to be piling on. Subtle changes make me feel less and less attractive. For instance, I no longer buy pants with zippers because my expanding mid-section just won't allow for them anymore. If there was a church that worshiped the invention of elastic waist pants, I would join immediately. There you would find me, the chubby one in the front pew praising St. Elastic, the patron saint of menopausal belly fat.

Oh, and bonus points for back fat! That's almost worse. The back fat makes it impossible to find a bra that both fits well and is comfortable. I am constantly scouring the internet for hints on how to hide my bulging waist. I now own my fair share of tunic tops and single-breasted blazers. It's expensive, time consuming, and annoying to have to focus on myself like this.

I live my life these days navigating this new world of ill-fitting clothing and fighting debilitating depression triggered by how unattractive I feel. When I think about hosting a party or even attending someone else's, I am immediately overwhelmed with what to wear and I usually decide to just stay home. I'm not sure what I'm going to do to change the numbers on the scale, or—more importantly—the way I feel about my body.

Meet Carol

Carol is a fireball. A natural born organizer who is very active in her community, Carol signs up for every "fun-run" and "walk for a cause" event to both support the city she loves and keep her body fit. Those who know Carol (and that seems to be just about everyone) would say she is extremely active and energetic. Lately though, Carol is becoming increasingly aware of changes in her menopausal body. No matter how much she exercises, her body just isn't responding in the same ways.

Story

I love to exercise. Most days, you can find me in a yoga class or running my daily five on the treadmill. I take a weekly exotic pole dancing class, which has really built my inner core strength and I feel especially sexy doing it! I believe in the value of moving my body and exercising. I like to stay busy.

For years I've played tennis, even playing on a woman's traveling team competitively for a while. Last year, I challenged myself with a new activity—riding and participating in a 3-day, cross-state biking tour, all with a group of people that I didn't know. We slept in tents and ate from chow wagons. I felt brave and gutsy and oh, so young! The next thing on my list is to get ready for the annual Michael Jackson's Thriller dance with a group of people from my city. It is such a hoot to watch people dress up like zombies and participate in this celebration of dance and community. You can find out more at ThrilltheWorld.com

Because of my focus on health and physical activity, my body has always been trim and fit—just about right for my height and bone structure. I usually can wear anything I want, even the new trends the teens wear. I never worried about bulges, muffin tops, or back fat. Until now, once I hit 45. It doesn't seem to matter what kind of physical activity I do, I keep gaining more weight. In fact, I've gained 25 pounds in the last two years, even though I have increased my physical activity.

It is so unfair.

When I look in the mirror, I now see my mother's body. My sagging breasts and ass, and an enormous amount of extra padding around my hips and stomach. Maybe worst of all is the thickening of my upper belly, right below my ribcage. This extra weight makes me feel old and unattractive and I feel disgusted with myself.

So, what's the answer? More exercise? No way. I'm maxed out on activity, and I cannot add another thing to my plate. I already work out five days a week for at least an hour. I sweat when I exercise too—I don't just phone it in. Still, the pounds keep piling on.

It really is so, so unfair. To find out more about worldwide event visit: ThrilltheWorld.com

Meet Mona

A reserved, quiet woman, Mona is happiest when creating a beautiful garden from seeds, conjuring up a fabulous meal with simple ingredients for her family of four, or designing and constructing a masterpiece quilt from discarded scraps of fabric. She stays busy with these activities she loves. However, quilting and cooking are not considered physical activities and as she moves through perimenopause, she finds herself gaining weight.

Story

I'm a dreamer. As a girl, I'd much rather curl up and read a book, or spend my afternoons water coloring, than going outside and playing. I did everything I could to get out of gym class and I much preferred sitting on the sidelines and cheering for my friends during ball games. As I now grow older, I spend my days gardening, sewing, painting, and movie watching. I have nothing in common with people who say they crave exercise. My cravings are around creating things, discovering things, and being with my family.

Speaking of cravings, I love to eat good food. My sons and daughter tease me about being a "foodie" and they're right! I love coming up with new recipes and I spend a lot of time buying the tastiest ingredients to serve my family each night. I'll admit it: I love pasta primavera more than taking a walk. I know I should exercise, and since I'm noticing my clothes getting tighter, I want to at least try. But because it's never been any kind of habit in my life, I don't know how to even start. A friend of mine suggests I try yoga, but I'm not sure my body would even begin to bend the way yoga seems to demand. All that downward facing dog... or cat... or cow... or crocodile... anyway, are you kidding me? And where do I even go for a class; what would I even wear?

I suppose I've got to do something, but I'm not sure how to re-focus.

Sip

Hormone Happy Hour

We all need a sparkling, happy drink when getting through this chapter. Weight gain is a heavy subject, so it's time to lighten it up. Let's shake one that will lift our spirits and celebrate all types of women, no matter where we are in our weight gain/loss/maintenance journey. I'm right there with you!

Sittin' Pretty Sparkle Martini

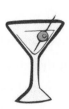
2 oz vodka or gin
2 oz prosecco
Three cinnamon red hots

This is easy and delicious! Gently stir the liquids together and pour them into a champagne flute. Drop three red hots into the bottom and watch them fizz. Just the right amount of cinnamon taste. Fizzy and pretty.

Sittin' Pretty Sparkle Mocktini

4 oz soda water
4 oz ginger beer (nonalcoholic)
Three cinnamon red hots

This is easy and delicious! Gently stir the liquids together and pour them into a champagne flute. Drop three red hots into the bottom and watch them fizz. Just the right amount of cinnamon taste. Fizzy and pretty.

Science of Why

Weight gain. The bane of the transitioning woman. Think of one of those creepy, scary fun houses that come to town with the fair. You enter one door, greeted with the mirrors that distort your body to maximum ugly; you shriek and run out of that room to enter the next, where the floors are tilted and you can't get your balance, and when you finally manage to stumble through the next door, gross, slimy monsters are jumping out at you... by the time you reach the end, you are exhausted, and there is no "fun" left in the experience. That is what it is like to research and study and really find out the Science of Why women gain weight during this time in their life. There are many different reasons, and they play off one another like a well-tuned orchestra. Are you ready? I wish I could say it is good news. It is not.

Fun House Door Number One – Increased Appetite

Like a teeter-totter on the kid's playground, as hormone levels decrease, appetite may increase-up to 50% more. In fact, studies using monkeys show during perimenopause and post menopause, when hormones are low, appetite may increase 76%–yikes (1)! Please let me not be like the monkeys.

More appetite = More eating = More weight gain

Fun House Door Number Two – Reduced Activity

Many women get complacent, or we feel entitled as we age (to relaxation, to sitting in front of the TV after a long day, to eating and drinking whatever we want–you know, we deserve to relax, don't we?) and so activity is reduced. Hormone imbalance can also decrease energy, leading to decreased activity. It is no secret that for many women, the majority of our work lives are spent sitting on our backsides, in meetings, in front of computers, in transportation. If we don't move it when we can–fitting it in before, during, or after our workday–the pounds will pile on (2).

More sitting = More weight gain

Fun House Door Number Three – Loss of Muscle Mass

We women need muscle. Muscle makes us look svelte and strong. Muscle uses more calories when working or resting than fat does. More muscle sends your body into a higher metabolism–meaning you will burn through more calories even at rest, and you will be more efficient in using calories, so they won't stay around and be turned into fat on your body.

Unfortunately, we lose an average of ½ pound of muscle mass a year if we don't preserve it with weight training exercise—and about 6.6 pounds per decade (3). What?! Yes, if you do nothing, you will lose muscle mass, and muscle mass is what keeps our metabolism humming to burn more calories—which is what we want. So, when you are sitting watching that favorite show, or driving in traffic, or working at your desk for hours, or even sleeping, your body is not burning up the calories you ate and drank all day like it could. The calories then get parked, on our bellies, our thighs, our hips, you know the drill.

Less muscle mass = Lower metabolism = Less calories burned.

Fun House Door Number Four – Calorie Intake

A twin challenge to the drop in metabolism is the fact that as our metabolism drops, we don't adjust our calorie intake. You know: eat less of the high calorie, low nutritional foods; drink less empty calories in sodas, coffees, and alcohols. Pair this with all you learned about food cravings, and this cycle can seem viciously hard to get out of. We want more, but should consume less. It can feel like, What do you mean? Just as I've reached a stage in my life where I am working hard, taking care of others, going through emotional highs and lows, and am experiencing more food cravings, it seems I should be able to eat and drink whatever I want, whenever I want. But no—now I have to also monitor my food intake. Damn! That seems unfair. And yes, dear friends, it is unfair.

Eating more of dense nutritional foods, like fruits, vegetables, and nuts, and less of the empty calorie foods, is essential to keep the creeping weight at bay. With a decreased metabolism and decreased amount of estrogens, we simply need less calories to stay at a normal weight (4). If we do not take care with caloric intake during perimenopause and menopause, studies show we are likely to put on at least one extra pound a year during our 40s and 50s, leading to 10-15 pounds of extra fat–just because (5)! Please, dear god...

Drop in metabolism + No calorie decrease = Weight gain

Fun House Door Number Five – Genetics

If you happen to carry genes that lend themselves to weight gain and obesity, it is doubly unfair (6). Genes help determine where we carry the weight on our bodies too. For example, some of us have saddle bag thighs, or a rounded pear shape, and some carry extra weight up in the chest and ribcage area. The thing about genetics is we can't change them, but we can still make choices to help ourselves. How our genes influence and affect our lives is complex, and a one-size-fits-all solution does not exist. As with any health-related issue, being professionally evaluated by a medical professional, and following sound advice concerning your body, and your genetic make-up is key to your health. Diet and exercise will always be a part of the equation, but there are other modalities that your body may need in order to be healthy. Honor your body and honor who you are. Arm yourself with knowledge and you will have more power to make positive choices for yourself, whatever your genetic make-up. There are many things we can't control in this life, but the key is focusing on what we can control.

Genetics do not dictate our being = Freedom to choose

Fun House Door Number Six – The Adrenals and Cortisol

By now you must be reeling from all the good news about weight gain. Ha! Keep going, I warned you it was not very good news. A conversation about weight gain is not complete without discussing your adrenals, what they do, and how they affect you. You've heard of Adrenal Fatigue? While this is not something you can get a medical diagnosis for, the collection of symptoms is real. The body experiences adrenal fatigue when you are under constant, unrelenting stress. This can be internal or external stress—it may come from your job, your family, your internal conversations, or the way you view your world and life. And why are we talking about adrenals here, in the weight gain section? Because what happens in the adrenals highly affects the way your body metabolizes calories and stores fat.

Your adrenals are small, walnut-sized glands that sit atop your kidneys. Their function is to help the body through stressful times by releasing adrenaline and cortisol, the hormones that help you manage stress. Adrenaline is fast acting—it's responsible for your pounding heart, breaking out into a sweat, and speeding your breathing up. It dictates all the immediate reactions you have when confronted with a new stressor, like seeing your dog almost get run over after she darts away from you into traffic, or an internal office memo you receive stating that job cuts are to be made during that day's newly scheduled afternoon meeting.

Cortisol takes a little longer to respond, but its release triggers energy to be freed from cells, so you are prepared to deal with the stressor. You have heard the example many times, that as early human beings, we needed the cortisol release in response to stressors so we could fight or run from predators—the fight or flight syndrome. When the body perceives danger or stress, our heart rate speeds up, the adrenals dump adrenaline and cortisol into our bloodstreams, and we can respond to the stressor.

However, when stress is unrelenting, and the stress is not the kind that demands our bodies exert physical energy, all that extra cortisol enhances the glucose (sugars) released into our bloodstream. If you have extra "fuel" coursing through your veins and you don't need it, that sugar or glucose converts to FAT—the padding many menopausal women see increasing on their abdomen, under the ribcage, around the back, and on the hips, inner things and stomach. Another consequence is something called visceral fat, the fat that packs around our organs deep inside the body. ACK! Unrelenting stress is a fat gain magnet.

Unless it's the kind of stress where you are fleeing from a predator, you don't need that extra glucose, so the body stores that glucose as fat.

Unrelenting stress = Increased cortisol = Increased blood sugars, not being used up = fat

"Adrenal fatigue" sets in when the combined, unrelenting stress overwhelms the body's capacity to regulate the cortical levels and it just keeps getting dumped into the blood, activating sugars that you don't use up. Metabolically, you are making too much fuel, and the body stores that fuel as fat. At the same time, the adrenals are working non-stop and overtime to meet the demands of the unrelenting stress, so you are constantly tired and overall fatigued. You can't get your energy up, you drag all the time, you basically feel like sh*t. Getting ahold of the stress in your life and learning to manage it is essential.

With all of the Fun House fabulousness of aging women, we do need some relief, some answers, and some hope that all is not lost to wobbly, widening weight gain.

Strategy

Tips for Living Your Best Self

Since the weight gain during menopause is multi-factorial, there are many things we can do to feel better and live better. The Fantastic Four play a huge role in weight maintenance, so be sure to thumb through that section again as well as following these tips.

Tip # 1: Support your adrenals

Help is on the way! We've got to get some support for our over-worked adrenals so they can play out their role in stress reduction and weight management. Two things we all want and need. Let's look at diet and lifestyle choices we can make to support them.

Cut out hydrogenated fats. When you take a normal fat, like butter, and force chemical hydrogen into it, (which allows it to stay hard at room temperature), that's hydrogenated fat. It is difficult for the body to breakdown and metabolize hydrogenated fats, and your adrenals will suffer. Look for the words "partially hydrogenated oils" in the ingredients of the foods you eat. Some common culprits are cakes with frosting, biscuits, frozen pizza, (the dough), microwavable breakfast sandwiches, and doughnuts (7). Eat whole foods, not those that are pre-packaged and filled with ingredients you can't even pronounce. Eat good fats instead, like olive oil, avocados, coconut oil, and nuts.

Reduce refined sugars. But it's so sweet and yummy. Yes, but refined sugars not only negatively affect adrenal health, they contribute to inflammation inside your body. Almost all chronic disease is inflammatory in nature, and we don't want to feed that. If you reduce the hydrogenated fats in your diet, you will go a long way in reducing sugars as well, as they often go hand-in-hand.

Reduce caffeine and alcohol. Why? Because they rev-up the adrenals. This is part of why coffee or caffeinated soda is so important to many of us in the morning—it revs us up, gets us going. But too much, or drinking it all day, stresses the adrenals. Alcohol on the other hand, depresses the adrenal gland's action, inhibiting the adrenals in their work. The more alcohol you consume, the more depressed your adrenals get. We don't want that. Depressed adrenals make for more stress in your body, which in turn makes for more weight gain.

Eat quality protein. Whey protein, or meats that are raised without antibiotics and allowed to range or forage. These types of meats have greater abundance of Omega 3s, in the right balance, to support optimal health.

Get plenty of sleep. Get a load of this: research shows that one night of sleep deprivation can lead to a 100% increase in cortisol the next day. And levels are still elevated the next evening (8,9). See more on proper sleep hygiene in the Fantastic Four section.

Take a B vitamin complex. Your ideal vitamin should contain B3, B6, and B12. Zinc, vitamin C, and magnesium also support the adrenals.

Have a sense of humor! Laughter is proven to be a tremendous stress reliever.

Tip # 2: Exercise

Nearly every one of the Fun House reasons for weight gain—increased appetite, reduced activity, loss of muscle mass, caloric intake and decreasing stress to support your adrenals—are better managed and helped by our good friend, Exercise.

Exercise for stress relief and adrenal support.

Exercise for building muscle mass—counteracting the natural decline.

Exercise for controlling appetite—endorphins and feeling good help you make better decisions regarding food intake.

Exercise for increasing activity—get moving and you are taking positive steps to manage the propensity to gain weight.

We need stress reducing, muscle-mass stabilizing exercise activities, whether that is a brisk, heart-pumping walk, or yoga and pilates, or a swim in the pool. If you simply detest the thought of exercising, try to incorporate it into activities you do love. If watching TV or YouTube is your thing, buy some light weights and do standing squats, arm raises, bicep curls, or deep stretches while watching your favorite programs. Do you appreciate beauty in nature? Find a friend to walk with. If you prefer solitary activities like crossword puzzles or crocheting, make it a point to do some of your activity while standing up, rather than sitting the entire time.

I will say it again: to live well and beat the Hormone Groan, we must engage in physical exercise. Find what you like. Make a plan. Do it!

Tip #3: Monitor your food intake – work to decrease it

This is easier said than done, especially understanding that often the desire to keep eating is frequently hormone driven (see Chapter Seven on food cravings) and habit based. The truth is, our bodies do not need the same caloric intake in our 40s and 50s as they did in our 20s and 30s. My husband has a favorite quote: "In your twenties, you can eat the entire pizza, in your thirties, a few pieces of the pie, in your forties, best just to have one piece, and in your fifties—no pizza." The point being, as our bodies age and lose lean muscle mass, we need less fuel to feed it.

Tips to try in our quest to monitor and reduce caloric intake:

- Drink half your weight in ounces of water daily.

- Fill your plate with primarily vegetables, fruits, good carbs (whole grains, brown or wild rice, quinoa—any carb not derived from refined white flour), and a small portion of protein, then you can eat the whole thing. Lean proteins such as chicken, fish, eggs, and tempeh help the body feel full, so less calories are needed from low-density foods to fill you up (10).

- Whether your nemesis is chips or ice-cream, eat them only once a week.
- Stop eating after 7pm at night.
- Write down how much you are eating each day, or track what you eat in an app—this act often helps you eat less and keeps your mind focused on mindful eating. In fact, in a scientific

review published in the Journal of the American Dietary Association, "self-monitoring (of food intake) is the center-piece of behavioral weight loss intervention programs" (11). It works, people!

- Mind over matter. Engage your brain to be aware of what you are eating, to focus on positive affirmations regarding what you will and won't eat.

There are hundreds of programs out there to help you with knowing what and how much you are eating, with helping motivate you to get moving and stay active, and keeping you plugged in to your body's fitness and food needs. Find what works for you. I am a firm believer that there is no ONE WAY to lose weight and keep it off. I think pretty much any program will work if you work the program.

Take Action:

- **Keep track of what you eat this week.** Use an app, or good old pencil and paper. Pay attention to processed foods and fast foods. Decide what you could exchange in your weekly diet—for example, toss the morning store-bought muffin or pastries and exchange them for a piece of whole grain toast with avocado.
- **Examine your sleep habits.** Say no to doing more things in the evening so you can get the sleep you need to recharge and support your adrenals.

- **Pick up a complex B vitamin and start taking them daily.**
- **You know about exercise.** Plan it. Do it

There is no magic pill. Let that dream die. Sure, we can follow a diet regimen, inject ourselves with certain substances, drink shakes and teas, take all kinds of vitamins and supplements, get hooked on methamphetamine-type pills, but really, there is no secret to take away the propensity of gaining weight during perimenopause and post menopause.

The answer to the weight gain dilemma lies somewhere between accepting your new normal while taking care of and honoring yourself. Employing doable action steps can help you maintain a healthy weight and gain your personal power back. I work on this aspect of living and loving my life daily. Come join me in making positive changes to beat the Hormone Groan of increasing back fat and jelly rolls.

Chapter Nine

Mouth on Fire

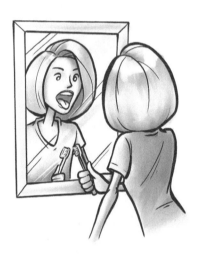

Meet Teresa

My name is Teresa and I am a pediatrician. My day typically starts when the alarm jolts me out of bed at 5:30 am. I stumble to the bathroom, pee, and brush my teeth. I can't stand morning breath—on me or anyone else. Gross! I stumble downstairs to hit "start" on the coffee machine and let the dog out. Those few moments of dark and quiet before the kids get up, before I've even looked at my phone, when I am sipping hot, heavy, sweet, coffee, are some of the best of any day. 'Cause once the family is awake, it is non-stop go go go to get everyone where they need to be and for me to get to my office on time. You know the drill. Recently though, I am experiencing some unpleasant symptoms in my mouth. As a pediatrician, I am aware that the mouth is a window to what is going on in the rest of the body, so I am more than curious to find out just what is going on here.

Story

My teeth and mouth have always been very important to me. I like them clean and white, and my breath smelling minty fresh. When I was younger and dating, I never had less than two packs of gum, floss picks, and those tongue scraper deals in my purse at all times. My car was also always stashed with a pint of minty-fresh mouth rinse in the glove compartment, along with an emergency toothbrush and floss. These habits have carried over and are now just part of my life.

I know, I know, lots of people don't like to floss, but I do. It's actually kind cool to flip the food gunk out from between my teeth and watch it fly! But the worst thing is to leave it all in there, lurking between my teeth–ROTTING between my teeth. Did you know that food can rot in there? Sometimes I smell people's breath, and you can just tell there is rotting food in their mouth–GROSS! That will never be me, 'cause I am a bit anal about keeping my breath fresh and mouth clean.

I wish everyone was. Being a pediatrician, I see kids of all ages, and parents, all day long. In my office, I make sure we address good oral health habits, along with the whole health of the patient. I council mothers with newborns and infants how to gently wipe out their baby's mouth after they've nursed or had a bottle. I have my staff show the younger children how to swish-and-spit with their favorite mouth washes and brush their teeth; we even have a "mouth cleaning station" in the office, stocked with toothbrushes, toothpastes, and rinses.

So, I was alarmed and somewhat pissed last week when I discovered my gums were red and inflamed and started hurting when I was brushing. Then my tongue started burning one evening while I was drinking my favorite red wine. That silky, full mouth feel I wait for as I sip the wine was gone. Instead, as the wine filled my mouth, my tongue felt like it was on fire. It was painful. I swallowed and tried it again...Yep, there was definitely a burning sensation on my tongue. Damn! How dare my mouth betray me and deny me one of the primary pleasures I look forward to all day long.

I then remembered I had experienced this burning while I drank my coffee in the morning. For the last few days, this had disrupted my zen time at the kitchen counter.

The following week, I went to my twice-yearly dental visit. I told my dental hygienist what was going on and as she examined my mouth, she said two things that alarmed me, "It looks like you are experiencing geographic tongue and some inflammation of the gums." WHAT!! What the hell is "geographic tongue"? She showed me some pictures of tongues that looked like a map of the world, then had me stick out my own tongue and looked in a mirror. Yep, there it was—my tongue had different areas where it was red and raised, no clear lines but rather like a topographical map where the mountains and valleys are different colors. WEIRD, and, how in hell could I have "inflammation of the gums"? I take meticulous care of my teeth. But I could see a red line around my teeth where they connect to the gums, and I had to admit, a couple of times this last month there had been a little pink color on my toothbrush after I brushed my teeth, which I now know was blood.

What was going on and why was this happening? My science-oriented medical doctor get-to-the-diagnosis-and-treatment part of me was on high alert.

Sip

Hormone Happy Hour

What's needed here, for you and Teresa, is a drink made to quiet and calm the mouth. Soothing green tea antioxidants and the anti-inflammatory properties of the coconut oil will have you peaceful and happy soon.

Green Coco Soother Martini

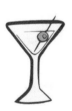

2 oz vodka

2 green tea bags steeped in 4 oz hot water

1 tsp coconut oil

Splash simple syrup or honey

Cinnamon stick

Steep one green tea bag in 4 oz of hot water for 5 minutes. Remove tea bag. Melt coconut oil into green tea. Stir in vodka. Add simple syrup to taste.

Serve warm in a beautiful glass with handle. Place the cinnamon stick cross ways over the cup for garnish.

Green Coco Soother Mocktini

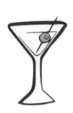

2 green tea bags steeped in 8 oz hot water
1 tsp coconut oil
Splash simple syrup or honey
Cinnamon stick

Steep two green tea bags in 8 oz of hot water for 5 minutes.
Remove tea bags. Melt coconut oil into green tea. Add simple syrup
or honey to taste.

Serve warm in a beautiful glass with handle. Place the cinnamon
stick cross ways over the cup for garnish.

Ahhhhh!! Soothing green tea antioxidants and the anti-inflammatory properties of the coconut oil will have you calm and happy soon!

Science of Why

First off, it's very weird that even the inside of your mouth could be
affected by perimenopause and after. I mean, can't we have one area
of the body that is left alone? Well, maybe you'll be the lucky one,
but many of us will experience changes here. Of course, the cause of
the changes have to do with your dropping hormonal levels, and the
hormone receptors in the mouth not being filled up. Yes, there are
estrogen hormone receptors deep in the cells of your mouth, just like
many other tissues within the body.

Remember the lock and key analogy? If the locks are not filled
with keys, changes in the gingiva and oral mucosa can happen. Wait
a minute, gingiva, and oral mucosa? Come on girl, you're talking
like a dental professional, get real. What is that? These are all the
surfaces on the inside of your mouth, the gums that surround each

tooth, your tongue, the inside of your cheeks, under your tongue, the roof of your mouth, all of it in there. The tissues inside your mouth are FULL of hormone receptors at the cellular level. When the receptors are left empty, changes can happen within the cells themselves, modifying how cells turn-over, how they become different types of tissues, and how they grow. All of this leads us to experience different symptoms and sensations in the mouth (1). The good news is, some of the changes are only episodic, or transitional, meaning the symptoms will diminish when the body gets used to the new level of hormones in the body.

And what can happen when the cells inside your mouth are changed? Read on for the fascinating details.

Increased dry mouth – The medical term is xerostomia. This is when your mouth is very dry, and it can feel sticky or gummy. Your tongue may feel like it doesn't work properly or sticks to the roof of your mouth, or like it takes extra effort to open your lips and get words out. All of this happens when you don't have enough saliva in the mouth. We need our saliva to keep the mouth moist and help the tongue work correctly when speaking and swallowing. It also plays a large role in keeping foods and sugars swept off the teeth. Many medications can cause xerostomia, but so can going through menopause. Dry mouth can lead to more cavities, mouth sores, fungal infections, and of course, bad breath. Yuck! Get me some moisture.

Increased risk for gingivitis – This is inflammation of the gum tissues, which is what our friend Teresa was experiencing. The gums become reddened. Especially right along the surface where the teeth come out of them, they bleed easily and are a little swollen. Your gums (gingiva) experience a change in their color and texture. The good news is gingivitis is reversible with good oral hygiene and self-care. More on that in the tips section.

Burning mouth syndrome – This is exactly as it sounds. A condition where the mouth feels like it's on fire! Some describe it as a burning or tingling sensation. In severe cases, it feels like your mouth is scalding—even when not partaking of hot or even warm food and beverages. The mouth can feel numb, and you may experience altered taste perceptions, where things taste more bitter or metallic.

Geographic tongue – Think "map." This is a benign, harmless situation where the top and sides of the tongue have areas of change in color and depth. Geographic tongue is considered an inflammatory disorder and often makes the tongue resemble a map. Sometimes it does cause change in taste perceptions, or feels like burning mouth syndrome. Your tongue is covered in small finger-like projections called papilla, and during an episode of geographic tongue, some of those papilla get blunted or lost, so the appearance of the tongue is changed. It often looks like areas of redder color which are slightly raised, causing the tongue to look like a map (2).

With both burning mouth syndrome and geographic tongue, the causes aren't entirely clear, but research does show that the perimenopausal woman may suffer from these conditions periodically, or off and on (3). Have you stuck your tongue out while in front of a mirror lately? Try it, and see what it looks like...If you know what your "normal" tongue looks like, it will be much easier to see if and when you experience any changes to it.

Altered taste perception – Suddenly your cheesy, gooey homemade macaroni casserole doesn't taste cheesy good anymore, and your chocolate chip cookies aren't sweet enough. With this condition, things taste differently than before—suddenly you can't taste the salt or sour or sweet. It may come as a result of burning mouth syndrome or geographic tongue, or it may not. In any case, it usually is episodic, and won't stay for long periods of time (4). Best to have someone else be your taste tester for a while. And, upside, if things don't taste as delicious, perhaps that will help you resist the goodies!

Increased risk of periodontal disease – First, what is periodontal disease? You read a bit about gingivitis earlier, which is inflammation of the gum tissues. Periodontal disease is when that inflammation is not disrupted or stopped, and simply put, bad bacteria are allowed to grow and set up house inside your mouth. Eventually, the bacteria and their by-products cause destruction of the supporting structures of your teeth, including the gums, bone and ligaments that hold your teeth in place. Think of it like the foundation of your house; if there are cracks in it, or it's shifting a bit, you may be able to get along with it like that for a while, but if you let it go and don't take care of it, eventually the whole house will start to crumble, list, fall, walls cracking, all the way into a dilapidated state where it has to be torn down. That's periodontal disease. It eventually destroys all the structures holding your teeth in your mouth, as well as negatively affects other body systems and disease states. Once the bone is gone, the disease is not reversible (5). You do not want to get periodontal disease for multiple reasons, including keeping your nice smile and sweet breath.

Changing hormonal levels are a key player in oral health, but so are the effects of stress, cortisol levels (remember the adrenals from Chapter Eight), and depression. The Journal of Periodontology (which is considered the Bible of Dentistry) has focused its research on these three and their effects on periodontal disease. We know that increased stress during this stage of life can be detrimental to other areas of change we are going through, like weight gain, sleep, and emotional health, so no surprise that it can also be a player in periodontal health and disease (6).

Strategy

Tips for Living Your Best Self

ACK!!! Give me some relief here! While we may not be able to avoid all of these symptoms within the mouth, there are some practical tips to help keep your teeth and gums fresh and healthy.

Tip #1: Practice good oral health habits daily

Prevention is always better than treatment. And most all oral disease is entirely preventable, so let's get on this clean mouth track where fresh breath and kissable mouths are the norm. Prevention 101 means thoroughly brushing your teeth at least twice a day, and cleaning in between your teeth after eating—floss or picks, a water-flosser or those handy interproximal and interdental cleaners. Find something you like, that works for you, and get the gunk out from between your teeth. Chew sugar free gum after meals or snacks if you can't brush, because the action of the chewing helps dislodge some of the food particles stuck in between the teeth and increases the saliva flow, which helps sweep out the mouth. Incorporate an oral health rinse into your daily routine to further strengthen teeth, and clear out the bad bacteria. This will work to prevent gingivitis and periodontal disease.

Tip #2: Use products that are SLS free, if needed

What is that? SLS stands for Sodium Lauryl Sulfate and is found in many toothpastes and mouth rinses. It is a chemical (considered a detergent and surfactant) that helps products foam. You know, that minty, fizzy foam that we have experienced most of our life when tooth brushing. SLS may denature or change the top layer of mucosa (all the linings in your mouth) causing pain and discomfort. Perimenopausal women are more highly reactant to detergents and surfactants in dental products, especially if you are suffering from geographic tongue or burning mouth syndrome. Also, if you are prone to getting canker sores, SLS can be irritating (7). So, if you are experiencing these conditions and symptoms, it is recommended that you use products that are SLS free. Google it—they are out there on your drugstore's shelf and easy to find.

Tip #3: Increase your intake of B12 vitamins

Research suggests that this may help block geographic tongue. Low levels of B12 can lead to changes in the tongue surface, so be sure to get enough B12 in your diet and/or supplements. Now, you want to know how much is enough, right? The recommended daily intake by the National Institutes of Health (NIH) is 2.4 micrograms a day but the Food and Drug Administration (FDA) sets the Daily Value at 6 micrograms (8,9). So somewhere in between those two are safe and recommended for most people. Unfortunately, you can only find out what your B12 levels are with a blood test. If you are suffering from geographic tongue, consider upping your intake of foods where B12 naturally occurs. These would be things like Atlantic wild salmon, turkey breast, eggs, milk, non-fat yogurt—or consider a Complex B vitamin supplement.

Tip #4 Reduce stress

Yes, this is important for your oral health. I could just cut and paste what I have already said about this in the book, things like support your adrenals, practice deep breathing, honor your senses and partake in sights, sounds and feelings that make you happy, use meditation to lower stress. It's kind-of like exercise, we need to work on it. Period.

Whew! Who knew so much could happen in your mouth during the menopause journey? It makes sense though, because there are hormone receptors in so many tissues throughout the body, your mouth included.

Take Action:

- **Examine your oral health habits, and make sure you are brushing at least twice daily.** Find what works best for you to clean between your teeth, and do that at least once a day, if not after every time you eat.
- **Check out your toothpaste and mouth rinse ingredient list.** Do they have SLS in them? If you are suffering from any of the above symptoms, like burning mouth or dry mouth, find SLS free products to replace them.
- **Do something every day to relieve your stress.** Set your mind on calmness and gratitude. Practice deep breathing.

Working to get your hormones in balance can also help alleviate some of the causes of oral health distress. Turn to the Fantastic Four to learn more about hormone replacement therapy.

Paying attention to your mouth and practicing good oral hygiene is really the best advice for you. Women in this age range are more susceptible to all of the above mouth-on-fire issues. If you are experiencing any of these conditions, it is also helpful to see your dental health professional. Grab a new toothbrush, take a look at the products you are using, and do something nice for yourself. You can beat this Hormone Groan.

Chapter Ten

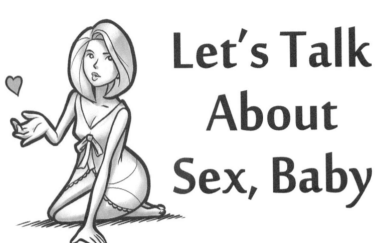

Let's Talk About Sex, Baby

Meet Mary

Mary is, by all accounts, a total sweetheart. She has always worked in the service industry: the sales counter at her local department store, intake specialist at a tire shop, and manager of a secondhand store. In each job, she strove to make the customer feel good, understand their needs, and bring a smile to their face. A few years ago, she went back to school and became a massage therapist. She lives to make people feel good, feel loved. A true romantic, the human connection is very important to her. Mary also has always enjoyed—no loved—having sex. Her sexual history is full of interesting and fulfilling encounters; she sees sex as an extension of the way she loves people and loves herself. Lately though, things are changing for Mary, and this menopausal pause in her sex life is causing her angst.

Story

I have always loved sex. Married young, while still a virgin, I couldn't wait to get to it. The way I was raised, marriage was the only way to get to sex. And once that door was opened to me, I never looked back! My first husband and I had sex often, and I loved everything about it, the sweat, the smell of his skin, the feel of our bodies' weight on one another...And I came easily, literally from the very first time we were naked together. Positioning myself so my clit got maximum exposure was important to me, and I loved the challenge of working to come together at the same time! Fun, explosive stuff!

When I divorced in my early thirties, dating was a whole new playground. Sex was part of the fun of the hunt, the chase, and the sharing. I no longer believed that sex was just for marriage, but that it was a measuring stick of compatibility, a natural part of the dating scene and getting to know someone more intimately. I was open about telling my partners what I wanted and needed and sex continued to be a big, happy part of my life.

Ten years into my second marriage, the same pleasure and release was part of every week. But in my late forties, things started to change. I could no longer orgasm consistently, which had always been my game. It wasn't even every time we hit the sheets, but some nights, nothing. No revving happened, no warm glow growing to sweet release, no tingling feel-good. Just nothing.

Just crazy thoughts I'd never had to deal with before like, "What is happening here?" "Come on body—get to it!" "Hurry up and get finished," "OH my god, let's just get through this for marriage maintenance!" Just feeling guilty and ashamed and angry when I wouldn't orgasm. My husband was patient and loving and doing all the right things; it just didn't seem to work anymore sometimes.

This was a huge change and loss for me. Loss in self-identity (if I couldn't orgasm, who was I sexually?), loss in pleasure, loss in something I truly loved to experience, loss of the release of those endorphins and the subsequent, total relaxation.

In addition to the lack of orgasm, sex was becoming painful. The very act of a rock-hard penis entering my vagina (which normally was a complete turn-on), felt like a burning metal rod going up inside me. This was putting a strain on my relationship, and dear god, I needed to find out what was going on? How could I get that crazy, feel good, screaming release back and enjoy sex again?

Sip

Hormone Happy Hour

We need a yummy concock-tion for this topic. Coconut water naturally is full of electrolytes and potassium, ingredients that are usually found in artificial sport drinks. And good sex is like a sport—it releases endorphins, causes your heart to race and skin to sweat. So, let's get ready to rumble and enjoy the release!

The Screamin' O Martini

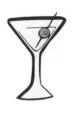

2½ oz vodka

1 oz coconut water

½ oz simple syrup

Lemon-lime soda

Half-n-half

3 Amareno cherries

Muddle two Amareno cherries with a teaspoon of its syrup. Add vodka, coconut water, and simple syrup. Shake thoroughly. Pour into chilled martini glass. Top with lemon-lime soda and a splash of half-n-half. Garnish with a cherry.

The Screamin' O Martini Mocktail

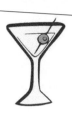

~~2 oz lemon lime soda~~

2 oz soda water

2 oz Coconut water

3 Amareno cherries

Half-n-half

Muddle two Amareno cherries with a teaspoon of its syrup. Add sodas and coconut water. Stir. Pour into chilled martini glass. Add a splash of half-n-half. Garnish with a cherry.

Science of Why

Gone baby gone, where did your love of sex go and will it ever return? Now, some of you reading this could care less if it returns or not—you are done with sex and don't mind the changes, don't miss it.

(And I'm going to get opinionated with you here. If you are done with sex, I encourage you to take another look, because sex has so many healthy consequences—it's good for your skin, your hair, your stress levels, and your cardiovascular system. Sex is good for you. I'd hate to have you give it up.)

Conversely, there are huge numbers of women out there who do enjoy sex, or did enjoy sex, like our pal Mary. You miss the intimacy, the releases, the sexiness you felt about yourself. Perhaps you are experiencing other symptoms of hormonal change and feel like your whole life is throwing one big wet blanket over sex.

It doesn't have to stay that way—you can get your sexual groove back, the strategies are coming. But first, let's look at the three main areas that women see sexual changes in: sex gets painful, your very sex drive and the desiring of sex changes, and negative body issues want to take the front seat (1).

Painful Sex

There are multitude of things happening through the body during perimenopause that affect the vaginal-vulva region. Don't you love that word? Vaginal-vulva? So sexy. We know estrogens are fluctuating up and down, surging, and waning. The vagina and the entire vaginal-vulva region is a very estrogen sensitive area. So if your body is not producing enough estrogens on any given day, and as you age, you make less and less estrogens, then your receptors may sit empty. One specific area full of estrogen receptors is the lining of the vagina. Estrogens in the vagina help create the natural lubrication and moistness of the area. If the vagina is dry, there ain't no technique that will bring back that loving feeling. This is why many women report that intercourse may become uncomfortable or painful, because the lining of the vagina is too dry and the tissue is too thin (another consequence of low estrogens).

Sex Drive Changes

Sexual response is how your body changes emotionally and physically during arousal and sexual activity. The heart speeds up, blood vessels open, your vagina gets wet and all the good, sweaty, I-am-so-hot-and-I-want-you-now stuff happens. This response has always been driven by desire for sex, and the sex drive itself. This is called the primary stage of sexual response. During menopause transition, the body is shifting that primary sexual response from desire to a place where sexual arousal or stimulation starts the revving of sex. As the sex drive wanes, sexual arousal, not sexual drive, becomes the primary force. Instead of starting with the I-want-you-so-bad drive, sexual response starts with all the arousal pieces of foreplay and emotional connection. So, as we age, the things that drive the sexual response change. Spending time and energy in creating sexual arousal and stimulating sexual zones becomes more important.

Besides the estrogens, we must talk about testosterone. This is primarily a male dominant hormone, but we women have it too. And we need it. Think of all the estrogens a woman has in her body as a full cup, while all of her testosterone fits into a small but important teaspoon. Besides helping us retain and grow muscle mass and contributing to bone health (both of which are super important as we age, testosterone drives sexual desire) (2). As our estrogens wax and wane and gradually drop, so does our testosterone, plunging our sex drive with it.

Body image issues

You know what this is...as our bodies change with age, we women tend to be very critical of them. Gone is the taught firm skin of our youth, and if you were lucky enough to have them, the tight ass and high perky boobs. Things shift, they sag, and often our size increases. Instead of loving ourselves, living our best selves, and embracing our new reality, we cover up, we shrink from intimacy, we think all sorts of negative thoughts about our worth, our value, our loveliness. If you have a committed partner close to your age, guess what? They are going through changes too. Be encouraged: our sexuality can be a normal, fun, satisfying part of our lives long past menopause. There is no age or body type that dictates when sex is over for us (3).

Strategy

Tips for Living Your Best Self

Let's look at all the positives things we can do to bring back that lovin' feeling.

So, hormones are dropping and changing, orgasms are few and far between, desire is...bleh...but you want it back. The steamy, I can't wait to get your clothes off, kiss me, touch me now! feeling.

The Fantastic Four play an important part in our overall sexual health. If you are eating right, exercising, and getting enough sleep, your life satisfaction will be higher, which plays a big role in affecting your sexual self. Hormone replacement therapy can be a positive game changer in the sex department. Read on.

Tip #1: Hormone testing and therapy

It's important to find a medical practitioner who gets women, who gets that our symptoms are real, and who can do thorough hormone testing. Perhaps you need a tiny dose of estrogen and testosterone. Perhaps you need more progesterone to balance out your estrogen. Every woman is different and thorough hormone testing will reveal your specific levels and needs. One sunny July, when I would normally be enjoying a healthy sex life with my husband, all of a sudden the desire was gone. I felt no need for sex, no want to, no passion. As this was a departure from normal for me, I went to my nurse practitioner who specializes in women's health to get my hormones tested. Sure enough, my testosterone levels had dropped "below the basement" she said. She recalibrated my bio-identical hormone prescription to increase the testosterone a wee bit, and within a couple of weeks, sex was again on the pleasure menu. Hormone therapy can help with the symptom of a changing sex drive.

Localized hormone therapy may also help if engaging in sex is painful (4). If the vagina and vulva area are dry, sex can hurt. Also, the tissues inside the vagina thin out as we age, so without enough moisture, the lining can get micro-tears in it. Ouch! An estrogen suppository can rev up that vaginal lining and get it ready for pleasure. It fills those estrogen receptors and supports the tissues themselves.

Balancing your hormones will make everything better, including your sexual self. Find a practitioner who can help you.

There are also tons of things you can do to get that engine revved and ready for pleasure that are non-hormone related.

Tip #2: Pleasure your senses

Indulge in things that bring you pleasure and make you feel sensual. Maybe it's reading erotica, stories that make your vagina get wet (or want to get wet), maybe it's watching porn, smelling your favorite candle, taking a warm bubble bath with a glass of wine, putting on silky underwear—anything that makes you feel sensual will help you in the bedroom. Listen to music that gets you feeling good. One of my favorite go-tos is an old K. D. Lang album, All You Can Eat. I mean, even the title is a turn on. Dim the lights, dance around with yourself or with your partner, and see what happens.

Tip #3: Use your brain

Thinking about sex can help your body want it more, and get ready for it. Notice others around you being sexual or flirting. Indulge in sexual fantasies. Read articles, or stories with sex in them, listen to pod casts about sex, remember positive sexual encounters and how good they felt. Where were you? Who were you with? You can go all out and recall every detail, or just let the memory wash over you and bring you pleasure.

Tip #4: Focus on your body

Especially if you suffer from poor body image. Time, again, to check the negative self-talk and focus on your body's positive attributes. Focus on being healthy in your body and mind—not a certain weight or body fat content. Living a healthy lifestyle with regular exercise, socializing with good friends, engaging in activities you like or that support your view of the world, are immensely important when it comes to sex. The better you feel about yourself, your body, and how you live, the better your sex life will be.

Tip #5: Talk about sex with your partner

Speak up! It is helpful to talk with your partner about what is working and what isn't. Perhaps the same habits of foreplay and intercourse need a change-up. Don't be afraid to experiment with new things: positions, toys, or sexual activity other than intercourse. Working on sexual communication becomes more important as our bodies change with maturity. If your partner is close to your age, or in that shifting place of 40-60ish, they too are probably going through some sexual changes. Whatever the age of your sexual partners—open, compassionate communication is key during these times (5).

Tip #6: Put sex on the calendar

I know this sounds like the antithesis of sexy, but setting the date and time for sex can be very helpful. For one, you can think about it and anticipate it. You can work your calendar so you are more likely to be ready for an orgasm, rather than hoping the whole thing will hurry up and be done because you are exhausted and have a million things on your mind. You could also schedule sexy activities, like shopping together for sex toys or lubes, exploring new ideas and products. Perhaps going dancing together makes you horny, or watching sex scenes in a movie. Whatever activities you do to enhance sexual pleasure—planning for sex gets you ready for sex.

Tip #7: Don't stop

There are so many positive health boosts you get from having sex. During sex, our bodies release many different hormones and elicit bodily changes that are good for you. Here is just a short list of the positive benefits you could gain from sex.

- Reduces chronic pain
- Exercises your heart
- Lowers breast cancer risk
- Lowers stress levels
- Powers up immune system
- Makes your heart pump harder
- Adds to vaginal health, plumps the vaginal walls, fighting against the dryness and thinning that can cause pain—sex begets healthy vaginas.

Tip #8: LUBE

One answer is lube, lube, and more lube! Get into the habit of using lube as a younger woman—younger meaning as you start to experience perimenopause, as this will totally save your bacon when you hit menopause and beyond, when estrogens are nearly non-existent.

A word about lubes: natural is better. Use a lube that has NO, read ZERO, sugars in it. I know the advertisements are hot and heavy with the lubes that taste good, smell good, and are intended to promote all kinds of oral sex, thus the taste good (which, I'm certainly not knocking the oral sex part, or even the taste good part). BUT anything with sugars in it is bad for women. Have you ever had a yeast infection? Lots of gross, smelly discharge gushing out of your sweet vagina. Uncomfortable and disgusting. And you have to get to a doctor, stat, for a prescription or it just lingers...Well, sugars are the preferred meal, snack, and sustenance of yeast. If you don't want yeast, you don't want sugars in your vagina. Another common ingredient in lubes is glycerin, which is similar to glucose (sugars) and can also potentially create that fertile breeding ground for bad bacteria, causing yeast infections.

Go to your organic food store and find a fragrance free, sugar free, natural lubricant. An excellent lube is plain old coconut oil. It has no additives, and is a natural anti-inflammatory. It even has a nice smell to it, and the tasting part, should that be where you're headed, is like a tropical pina-colada! (One note of caution: coconut oil may compromise the integrity of latex condoms, so if you are using those, beware too much oil.)

Tip #9: Self-love & masturbation

I cannot end an entire chapter on sexuality and not talk about masturbation as an act of self-love and a wonderful activity to help you navigate the changes you may be experiencing sexually. Many women were raised to think of masturbation as sinful or bad and dirty. We were told, "nice girls don't do that," if anyone spoke to us about it at all.

Fortunately, part of the beauty of reaching this stage in life is we can break free from negative thoughts and feelings about our own sexuality and engage in activities that feel good and are good for us. If masturbation is not an activity you regularly engage in, I encourage you to experiment and learn how to please yourself sexually. We then are not dependent on anyone else for our sexual satisfaction and release. Plus, the more you know what your body needs and likes, the better sexual partner you will be, if partner sex is part of your life.

I am a big proponent of vibrators.

While in grad school in my forties, I was carpooling with two other women, one in her early twenties, the other just into her thirties. The 30-something had a sexual habit of always using a vibrator to cum, before her boyfriend entered her and they got busy. Her vibrator worked so well for her that she rarely came with him inside her. She used it daily, whether he was around or not. The 20-something talked about not using a vibrator at all, she would just get-off using her own hands. Until that point, I had not ever used a vibrator (I was a little embarrassed to admit this, even to myself), and hadn't made myself orgasm without a partner since I did gymnastic stretches as a teenager.

My curiosity was so piqued by this conversation that I researched and wrote entire educational papers on sex toys, women, and masturbation, and presented them at regional conferences (6,7). But I felt I had no personal need, as my sex life was quite satisfying. However, my curiosity grew as I entered perimenopause, and started experiencing some changes, so I purchased my first vibrator. OMG! What was I missing all these years! Fast forward ten years from that time, and I have a travel version that goes with me on business trips, and my favorite toy lives next to my bed. Now, I can get that sweet, exhilarating release whenever I need it. And so can you.

Not having a sexual partner does not mean no sex. Getting older does not mean no sex. Learning to work with your own body and pleasure yourself is wonderfully empowering and healthy. You deserve the joy of mind-blowing orgasms, and masturbation can give them to you.

Take Action:

- **Use your brain to think about feel-good, exciting sex.** Discover what adds sexual thoughts to your imagination. Is it noticing people flirting, or having intimate contact around you? Is it reading certain books or webpages? Is it remembering a great sexual session? Pay attention to how it makes you feel.

- **Seek out and make an appointment to see a women's health specialist.** Work together to find out if hormone therapy, hormone vaginal supplements, or other treatments would help you get back that lovin' feeling.

- **Search out and purchase some organic coconut oil.** In a private time, use your fingers to put the oil on your clitoris and vaginal area. Feel how silky, slide-y good that feels. Explore yourself.

- **Cultivate an attitude of adventure and fun with your sexual self!**

The truth is, the sex drive does change during the perimenopause years, but sex can still be an important, healthy part of your life well beyond menopause itself. Your powerful brain and beautiful body, at this stage of life, can still "get it on" and enjoy sexuality. I highly encourage you to work with yourself, your partner (if you have one), and your medical provider to remain sexually active. With a little attention to yourself, and some revving up details, sex can continue to BLOW YOUR MIND!

Go Meno!

Ladies, I've loved sharing this journey with you. You have been my inspiration and motivation all along the way—women I've met while speaking at home and around the country, girlfriends and strangers who've shared with me your stories, your frustrations and your personal victories, and the ladies who show up at my Martinis and Menopause Soirees, sharing their excitement and creating with me such a supportive and caring community of women. Our Tribe. My Tribe. I thank you.

I wrote this book with the intention to help women—to help them understand what's going on in their bodies, help them not feel alone in their menopausal journey, and to put real do-able strategies into their hands, because the ultimate goal is to feel better, live better, and beat the Hormone Groan.

I hope that through this book, you've been able to see yourself in some of the women's stories and identify with what they have gone through. I hope that by this point, you've realized you aren't crazy, and that there are actual, physiological reasons for your menopausal symptoms.

I hope you realize deep in your bones that there is no shame in menopause, there is no shame in our aging bodies.

We are each unique, wise, and beautiful. Yes, we change and the change is real—but together we rise, as we all go through this journey together.

Knowledge is power. Now you understand the scientific reasons behind why you feel the way you do, and are equipped with an arsenal of real-life tips you can employ to work in your favor. Use the tools and tips that speak to you, the ones you know you need to incorporate in your daily habits and those you know will best support you.

I wish for you lowered stress levels, empowered habits, and tons of feel-good neurotransmitters. I wish for your body and brain to work optimally for you, and for you to feel fabulous about your unique, powerful self!

As for the martinis—let's not forget the importance of community, de-stressing, and sharing our lives with one another. Take the martini and mocktini recipes and shake them up with your friends and loved ones. Create new ones. Share together. Enjoy the experience, and try not to take it all too seriously!

I hope that these tools have increased your confidence and conviction to become your own health care advocate—finding practitioners who get you, people who love and support you, and drawing upon your own internal strength to beat the Hormone Groan.

I invite you to visit my website, www.kellijaecks.com, and share your stories with me there. I'd love to hear how you are navigating through this time of your life.

The good news is, the menopausal years are transitional—they will not last forever! Hang in there. Do not let the Hormone Hostage Zone define you—use your inner resources to stay empowered and energized through the transition, and create community with others going through the change right along with you. One day, you too will emerge victorious on the other side, feeling great again in your body and mind, strengthened with valuable knowledge and blissful FREEDOM!

No longer a hormone hostage, we can all stand tall and shout, "Go MENO!"

Fantastic Four

Living as our best selves means we feel good mentally and physically. Even through the ups and downs of changing hormones and the changing circumstances of our lives, we can all have superhero powers in beating the Hormone Groan by making small, do-able changes to our daily routines. In all my research and writing for this book, four areas consistently came up regarding how to eliminate or reduce many of the symptoms women face during the menopausal transition. Focusing on these four—Exercise, Food Choices, Hormone Replacement Therapy, and Sleep—will catapult you out of the Hormone Hostage Zone and into that wonderful space of living better and feeling better.

So here they are, the Fantastic Four: you can refer to them anytime depending on which symptoms you are struggling with. Disclaimer: I am not an exercise science major, a nutritionist, or a doctor. But I do know things that work—to keep us living better and free us from being a hormone hostage!

Fantastic Four # 1: The Queen of All – EXERCISE!

I know, I know, you hear it everywhere, how important exercise is to your heart, your bones, your brain, and your body. Exercise is good for EVERYTHING about you, including, you guessed it, all things perimenopausal. From hot flashes to brain fog to irrational emotions to weight management, exercise is the first line of defense to breaking free from the Hormone Hostage Zone.

Vigorous exercise is almost magical in what it does for us. Hang on there a minute—what is vigorous exercise you ask? Fair enough. Vigorous exercise means you are moving long enough and with enough energy output that you break a sweat. That can be walking at a pace just above leisurely for 30-40 minutes, or it can mean all out balls-to-the-wall cross-fitting, cycling, hot yoga-ing—you name it. It doesn't much matter what you do to sweat, only that you do it.

Almost magical? Yes, here is a short list of what vigorous (read sweaty) exercise does for us:

- Increases serotonin and feel good neurotransmitters: This helps with all the emotional side effects of menopause. The irritability, the sadness and depression, the out-of-control eating. You have read consistently in this book that we want as much serotonin, norepinephrine, and dopamine that we can get. Exercise helps your body and brain make more of those substances.
- Reduces severity of hot flashes: Exercise can balance out the lack of estrogens and can reduce hot flash severity by up to 75%.
- Reduces stress, improves your mood: We all need this, right?
- Decreases cortical levels: Too much cortisol results in increased belly fat, so decreasing those levels can have a positive effect on your waistline. Good news!
- Strengthens bones: Weight bearing exercise helps your body build stronger bones. Bone strength is a true concern as we pass through this stage into post-menopause. If we do nothing to maintain bone health, we will lose it.

- Increases better sleep: One of the other Fantastic Four. We all know how important sleep is and how our bodies crave it. Better sleep. Better life.
- Increase muscle mass: Gives us greater calorie burn at rest, yes please!
- Increases circulation: Your whole body will thank you—especially your brain, skin, and internal organs.
- Reduces risk of high blood pressure, heart attacks and strokes.
- Supports your adrenal glands: Which in turn lowers stress levels and allows your body to handle stressors more efficiently.
- Increases blood flow to your sexual organs: Setting you up for better, more satisfying sex.
- Tells your body to stay vigorous, vibrant and healthy. Who doesn't want all this great stuff?!

The honest truth is, not exercising is not an option as we age—we need everything from the brisk walk around the neighborhood to vigorous exercise where sweat is pouring off of you. Yes, pouring. The sooner you can wrap your head around that, the better off you will be.

The North American Menopause Society—the leading voice of menopause—states that, "Exercise may cause the same magnitude of change as that induced by estrogen therapy" (1).

Reaching for pills and replacements (which I am not discounting as they often are needed, and I use them myself, but I also exercise at least five days a week) before EXERCISE is like buying a European vacation package before paying your mortgage.

The fabulous thing about exercise is you can choose from so many types and activities:

- The yoga and pilates type classes that stretch and strengthen muscles, while helping to integrate your breathing with body action. This will release stress and help center your changing hormone and neurotransmitter levels.

- Aerobic exercise that gets your heart pumping will release endorphins that work to lower stress levels and increase the blood flow throughout your body and brain. Getting that heart pumping and those lungs breathing deeper will make you feel good mentally and physically.

- Weight bearing exercise is extremely important during the menopausal years to maintain muscle mass. Muscle uses more energy than fat, so the more muscle you build, the more energy, i.e. calories, your body will burn, even while in a resting state or during your normal daily activities. Weight bearing exercise also works positively on your bone health to protect your frame from osteopenia (low bone density) and osteoporosis (fragile, brittle bones) later in life. You want a tall, straight spine, and healthy bones to support your precious body. We must stress our muscles to maintain or increase our muscle mass as we age.

The truth is, once you find what works for you, getting your sexy sweat on feels so good. With your endorphins and feel good serotonin levels jacked up, you feel like you can conquer anything that comes your way. That high you get from working out and sweating cannot be replicated in a pill or hormone replacement supplements.

I have a couple of friends in their late forties and early fifties who do not exercise. Ever. They don't like to move, they don't like to sweat. Unfortunately, they are having some trouble with this change of life, with weight gain, depression and general negativity. And I would bet money their bones are suffering, along with their digestive tracts and their immune systems. Yes, exercise helps with all of those things too!

A few years ago, I had an "ah-ha" moment. I had always exercised to keep my weight at normal levels for my body frame and type. I exercised for my physical body and how it looked. As I entered perimenopause and all these changes started happening in me, I realized the exercise was as much for my mental health as physical, perhaps even more so. When I pull on my workout clothes and get to a class at the gym or go for a run in the park, my mood elevates, the world seems a better place, my irritation fades and I think good thoughts about myself like, "I am such a bad-ass!" and "I am so strong and fit!" This is the "ah-ha"—that exercise benefits my mental and spiritual health as much or more than my physical health. Even on days when I gear up and don't really feel like exercising, I encourage myself by thinking, "I am fighting heart disease, I am fighting cancer, I am making myself healthier by moving." It is a privilege to move, and a necessity if you are a perimenopausal woman.

Fantastic Four # 2: Food Choices

Food can be a super power for you, or the villain that pulls you toward the abyss. I am not a nutritionist, and don't pretend to be one, but there are proven truths we can all focus on to live better and feel better during this passage through life. What we eat has the power to affect us positively or negatively when dealing with many of the symptoms highlighted in this book.

So here goes:

First, we're going to talk about gut health. What? Yes, if your digestive tract is happy and healthy your physical and emotional life will be too. By GI health I mean eating and drinking things that support a healthy gut like whole grains, green leafy vegetables, fiber, fiber, fiber, plenty of water, and pro-biotics. What you don't want is constipation, diarrhea, or constant gas and bloating. If you suffer from these, you know what I'm talking about. These symptoms are not indicative of a healthy gut, and if you experience these often, you may need to see a gastroenterologist or do some food allergy testing.

For a start, pay attention to what makes your GI act up, and eliminate those foods from your diet. According the U.S. Food and Drug Administration the top eight food allergens are (2):

- Milk
- Eggs
- Fish (e.g. bass, flounder, cod)
- Crustacean shellfish (e.g. crab, lobster, shrimp)
- Tree nuts (e.g. almonds, walnuts, pecans)
- Peanuts
- Wheat
- Soybeans

You may not have full blown allergies to a food, but if it causes your throat or skin to itch or swell, or your GI to bloat and create unpleasant gas, you probably have a sensitivity to the food and it does your body no good to eat it.

Unfortunately, many times the foods you love the most are the ones your body does not digest well. You know, when you eat that greasy, yummy processed meat, gooey, cheesy, thick, white doughy-crust pizza, and call it vegetables because of the red sauce? And then you and all those around you regret it for the next few hours as your body tries to digest that slug of wheat and fat, tries to pull any nutrition it can from that pizza...and you are bloated, uncomfortable, and making multiple trips to the "elimination station" in your house. That is your body telling you that that food is not good for you. Start to pay attention to what your gut is telling you.

Case in Point: Both my daughter and I love to eat crusty, white, sourdough bread, ripped off the loaf, and soaked in olive oil, balsamic vinegar, and salt. We can devour an entire loaf in one sitting, easily. She lives across the country from me, so when we get together and have that rare opportunity to just hang together and relax, we will often go to the store and buy the crusty, just-baked loaf. We'll sit and talk, or power-up our favorite Reality TV cooking/travel show and tear into the bread. But both of us will regret it. Within the hour, our stomachs bloat—that kind of swelling where your pants have to unbutton, where you can actually see the belly rise until you feel five-months pregnant, and then the uncomfortable, sometimes painful gas bubbles get gurgling around in there. And when it comes time to eliminate that gas, no one wants to be around us, and we can hardly stand ourselves. Why do we do that? Every time we succumb to that sourdough siren, we regret it and vow to not pay that price again. Just like you, I must pay attention to what my gut tells me about what I eat and drink.

The gut, or small and large intestines, has a whole system of nerve endings called the "Enteric Nervous system," or the little brain. This enteric system creates 90% of the serotonin in your body. Serotonin is also produced in the brain as a feel-good neuro-transmitter. Gut serotonin works on your immune system so you are physically healthy, and there is all kinds of research happening now to determine how gut-serotonin plays a role in depression, mood swings, and brain health (3, 4). We do know that the gut serotonin communicates with the brain, convincing it to make more brain serotonin, and really, you want all the serotonin you can get, wherever it comes from, the gut or the brain.

The National Institute of Health does state that poor diet is a risk factor for depression; thus, a healthy diet may prevent depression (5). And what is a poor diet? You know the answer to this: a diet full of highly processed foods, fast foods, white sugars, white flours, heavy on red meat and fatty meat, and low in all the good things like fresh fruits and vegetables, good fats, whole grains, and lean meat. And the great news is, these kinds of healthy foods are what make a healthy gut! And a healthy gut leads to healthier emotions. And you KNOW that emotions are highly affected during the perimenopausal years.

Probiotics: I am a big believer in taking probiotics to keep your gut full of good, beneficial bacteria. Look for one that is made from live cultures. I take pro-biotics when I feel my gut is out of balance, usually during and after a holiday, with all the added sweets and different kinds of foods available. When I am traveling I take them, as this again is a time when my eating is not normal. All those conference lunches and client dinners eating out is a huge departure from what and when I normally eat when at home. Probiotics are especially important if you need to take antibiotics for any reason. The antibiotics will kill the bad bacteria in your gut, along with all your good bacteria, so you need to replenish the good stuff. Probiotics are essential for proper food absorption, nutrition, and general gut health (6).

Fiber: According to the American Heart Association, the average person needs 25-30 grams of fiber a day, and that is sometimes hard to get in our diets. The American diet only averages 15 grams a day, well below the recommended amount (7). This is due to a variety of reasons, but much is attributed to a diet of fast food in the grab and go culture we live in. Highly processed foods have little fiber. So, the more foods you eat in their natural state the more fiber you will get from your food. Still, it is tough to get all the fiber we need from food, especially when you consider that one cup of broccoli only gives you 5.1 grams of fiber, and who wants to eat three cups of broccoli a day? Not me. But there are a ton of natural foods that give you good fiber. For instance, one-half of an avocado can give you 6-7 grams; one cup of oatmeal can give you 4-5 grams, and one cup of black beans or lentils gives you a whopping 16 grams. There are a ton of websites out there to give you the breakdown of how much fiber is in what, so go ahead and google it up. Plus, there is an entire "health food" industry full of supplements, shakes, and pills that can help you get the fiber you need for health. Take the supplements you need after you work to eat real food for fiber.

Omega 3s: The importance of Omega 3s to the women in transition cannot be overstated. Remember our good friend serotonin we just talked about in the gut? Well Omega 3s are a strong serotonin enhancer. They help your brain create more. You want as much of that "feel good" brain neuro-transmitter as you can get. Omega 3s are considered essential fatty acids that work at the cellular level. Many of the symptoms dealing with moods, like irrational irritation and anger or sadness and depression, can be helped by adequate Omega 3s. While we won't get into the detailed science of how Omega 3s interact at the molecular level to bring balance to our brains and bodies—just know this: YOU NEED THEM. Your body cannot manufacture them on its own, so it's vital that you take them in either through food or dietary supplements (8).

So how do we get more Omega 3s?

The types of foods you want to be eating are these:

- Flax seeds, chia seeds, and their oils
- Seafood, especially fatty fish like salmon, tuna, mackerel, halibut, trout, oyster
- Nuts, especially walnuts
- Soybeans
- Vegetable oils like olive and coconut
- Green leafy vegetables, like spinach, kale, and broccoli
- Dietary supplements

Research shows eating fish high in Omega 3s has a protective benefit to the brain, and in general, people who consume Omega 3s in fish and fish oils suffer from depression less. Most of us will benefit from a supplement because we don't eat enough fish per week. Look for a supplement of Omega 3 at 1000-1200 mg a day, and if it is paired with DHA, the bio-availability of the Omega 3s is enhanced in your body. Pair that with eating whole grains and lots of fresh produce for your optimal Omega 3s. You'll feel so much better!

Complex B vitamins: Complex Bs give you energy, can clear the fog in your brain, help with depressive feelings, and make you feel alive again. A must if you are suffering from "feeling low." The B6 and B3s will up your serotonin levels by helping your brain hold onto and convert a substance called amino acid tryptophan to serotonin, which as you know by now, is hugely important in mood regulation (9). B12 plus folic acid are needed to make more norepinephrine and dopamine, the other feel good neurotransmitters. So up your B-complex and see the dark days lifting.

Caution: if you already are taking a prescribed antidepressant or anti-anxiety medication, you need to check with your medical provider first before taking these neurotransmitter enhancers.

Now you want to know how much B complex is enough, right? The recommended daily intake by the National Institutes of Health (NIH) is 2.4 micrograms a day, but the Food and Drug Administration (FDA) sets the Daily Value at 6M micrograms (10). So somewhere in between those two are safe and recommended for most people. You have to get a blood test to tell what your levels of B12 are.

You can get B vitamins from foods as well. These would be things like Atlantic wild salmon, turkey breast, eggs, milk, and non-fat yogurt. There are multiple websites that can give you ideas and details about where and how to get more B vitamins from food (11). Most of us will need to eat Vitamin B rich foods and take a supplement to get enough of the feel good, energy producing building blocks.

Vitamin D: Known as the sunshine vitamin, we want to get all of this one that we can. Research shows that Vitamin D levels and depression go hand-in-hand; the relationship goes both ways, one affects the other, like the chicken versus the egg example. Those with depression and suffering from feelings of sadness are usually also low in vitamin D. And conversely, those with low vitamin D levels are at a greater risk of developing depression (12,13). Um...no, thank you. Take a vitamin D supplement. How much, you ask? Depends on who you ask, but in my experience the 600-800mg usually recommended are too low. I recommend 1-5k a day as you work to lift your mood and support your brain health. My practitioner has had me on as much as 10k a day for months at a time to lift my levels. I live in a part of the country that does not get sunshine all year round and I need the supplementation.

There are many other supplements out there that claim to help with depression, or serotonin production. The list is exhaustive and everchanging; however, if you can up your intake of Omega 3s, B Complex, and Vitamin D, I can almost guarantee that you will feel better, have more energy, and enjoy a more positive outlook.

The Fantastic Four #3: Hormone Replacement Therapy

Consider getting tested and taking bio-identicals.

In the midst of controversy and two very distinct sides of an argument, I'm taking a stand. Bio-identical hormones changed my life, literally, and added to its quality as I navigated nearly ten years of menopausal transition.

Now that we've opened up the subject of hormone replacement, some education is in order. For most women, traditional hormonal replacement therapy will not be prescribed until late in the menopausal transition, because traditional medicine uses a blood test to measure your FSH (Follicle Stimulating Hormone) which shows the levels of FSH your body is producing. FSH is produced in the brain by our pituitary gland, and helps control menstrual cycles and the release of eggs by the ovaries.

You may or may not be successful in getting an FSH test, and you may not be prescribed anything. An elevated FSH level combined with not having a period in twelve months generally gets you the distinct designation of reaching menopause. Woohoo! Break out the champagne and throw the tampons away! But again, this doesn't necessarily mean you will be prescribed anything—which isn't very helpful to the tens of thousands of women needing something NOW.

Women who experience early menopause due to ovarian or uterine cancers, or certain surgeries, will be put on hormone therapy right away. This is to protect the body as it ages, when we need estrogens, progesterone, and some testosterone in order to keep bones, breasts, brain, and other tissues healthy.

Before bio-identicals, you may remember the great scandal regarding traditional hormones. These first hormone replacements were manufactured from isolated estrogens found in pregnant mares' (yes, female horses) urine, and our mothers and grandmothers were fed this stuff as hormone replacement (14). This hormone replacement was mostly prescribed for POST-menopausal women, not those going through the transition.

Studies were done. As it turns out all that "natural," i.e. horse urine, hormone replacement had some very negative results, like increased risk of cardio-vascular disease and stroke, no benefit to bone health, increased risk for breast cancer, endometriosis, uterine cancer, etc. (15). Bottom line, the study sought to prove the benefits of this horse-urine hormone replacement, and ended up proving how negative and even dangerous these hormones were. Women across the globe stopped their therapies and went cold-turkey.

However, that is not the end of the story.

Recent research emphasizes that it is beneficial to have hormone replacement DURING these transitional years and after menopause. There was a huge study done recently on women's health across the nation focusing on the natural history of midlife, including the menopausal transition.

For any science geeks out there, (if you are not a science geek, skip to the next paragraph—really, this is just not that interesting to a lot of folks) there is a Multi-site Longitudinal Study funded by the National Institutes of Health called the SWAN study. The study is co-sponsored by the National Institute on Aging (NIA), the National Institute of Nursing Research (NINR), the National Institutes of Health (NIH), the Office of Research on Women's Health, and the National Center for Complementary and Alternative Medicine. It was started in 1994 and is ongoing. It is legit. You can read more about it here: www.swanstudy.org/about/about-swan/

The results of the SWAN study concluded that estrogen replacement therapy is beneficial to the brain prior to perimenopause. In years past, estrogen was only prescribed to women post-menopause. So, during these premenopausal years, it is likely that some women will need estrogen replacement to not only protect bones and brawn, but the brain itself. There are over 300 tissues within the body that have estrogen receptors, including the brain. We need estrogen, or estrogen-like substances, to fill those receptors for the brain to function optimally. This is why it's important to be informed and empowered with what's happening in your body, so you can make any necessary changes or supplementations to support your best health.

Now, we need to talk about bio-identicals, what they are, what they can do, and where you can get them.

Bio-identicals are hormone-like substances created in a lab which have an identical chemical structure to a hormone produced in the body. They are usually (but not always) derived from plant substances, and act like a lock and key for hormone receptors in the body. As the bio-identical is floating through your blood stream, it finds the hormone receptor and locks right in, allowing your vital bodily functions to continue as they should.

After that debacle of the traditional horse urine-derived hormone therapies came the rise of the bio-identical, and the great debate. There are conflicting sides and opinions from all sorts of health and wellness players, including drug companies, the FDA, pharmacists, and natural products industries.

Part of the hoopla came down to this: drug companies cannot patent a plant-based substance, so these plant–based bio-identicals don't go through the FDA approval system. In this country, no FDA approval equals no oversight to test the effectiveness and ability of the substance to do what it claims it will do. So essentially, if you use plant-based bio-identicals, you have to be willing to take that risk.

Most plant-based bio-identicals are customized by compounding pharmacists. The pharmacy profession is regulated by state boards, so the FDA has no way to measure or control the compounded substance. On the flip side, each state pharmacy board does regulate and oversee the compounding pharmacists within its jurisdiction.

To add even more confusion to the mix, the FDA does now have approved bio-identicals made from chemical compounds (not plant-based.) These bio-identicals have gone through FDA approval; however, they are more of the one-size-fits-all prescription nature.

My journey to get bio-identicals started in my early forties, while I was in graduate school. My days were filled with researching, writing, teaching, grading, using my computer in ways I hadn't before, and using it for hours and hours at a time. I would sometimes be sitting at the keyboard, thick into writing a paper, when my mind would just go blank. I couldn't think of what I was going to type next; I would feel enveloped in fuzz. So yes, I was experiencing brain fog. And the simplest things my kids would say or do set me on edge. I had episodes of becoming the bitch mom I strived so hard not to be, yelling, stomping through the house, slamming doors. These explosions did not jive with my ideas about myself, and I found myself apologizing over and over. But one day in particular stands out—I was just finishing my first year of grad school, had written countless papers and assignments, and was well on my way into my thesis research and writing. Back in the day, our family only had one computer. I would use it for all my school projects and my teenage son would use it for gaming. He was a big gamer and I thought it was such a cool world for him to be a part of. That day, I was home alone trying to finish a writing project when the computer screen went black. I immediately panicked and emotionally went from calm and quiet to a RAGING, screaming lunatic! I completely melted down, crying, yelling, stomping, and throwing things. And while this computer shut-down was a big problem, my reaction to it scared me. I was out of control.

I knew I needed hormonal help and I went searching for it.

I found a nurse practitioner specializing in women's health and never looked back. Although I had medical insurance, her services, the hormone testing, and the prescriptions were not covered. Paying out of pocket for this was entirely worth it for my mental, physical, and emotional health.

Through testing, she prescribed bio-identical hormones individualized just for me. I would go in once or twice a year to be tested again, depending on how my body was reacting to life. With updated tests, I would get an updated prescription. Again, just for me, and what my body needed at the time. This work to keep my hormones balanced while my body transitioned to menopause was a life-saver. It helped with many of the symptoms described in this book, the emotional irritations and sadness, brain fog, hot flashes, changes in sexual desire, and my very energy to get up each day ready for whatever the world brought my way.

I also found relief through a progesterone-like bio-identical cream I purchased over the counter at my local natural food store. I rubbed a quarter-sized amount into my skin twice daily, and man, did it take the irritated edge off and help my brain concentrate. After a few months, my children and husband would notice if I wasn't on the cream because of my increased irritability and forgetfulness of the smallest, most normal things. Bio-identicals saved me during this time, and they're always the first thing I recommend to women just starting to experience the Hormone Groan.

The most reliable way to get a correct dosage and prescription just for you is to get a medical professional to prescribe you a bio-identical after hormonal testing. The prescription is detailed to your needs, with a specific dosage of estrogens, progesterone, and testosterone. This script is then made/filled by a compounding pharmacy.

How do I get a bio-identical prescription just for me?

In these last ten years, you would think it would be easier to obtain an individualized prescription for bio-identicals. The best tip I can offer is to find the compounding pharmacy nearest to you, call them up, ask for a list of medical practitioners who prescribe bio-identicals, and use their pharmacy. Then, get an appointment with one of those practitioners. (Keep in mind you may see an NP, naturopath, or chiropractor instead of an MD.) A great resource is to visit the International Academy of Compounding Pharmacists: www.iacprx. org—click on the "find a local compounding pharmacy" connection button under About on the homepage.

Find them. See them, get tested. Get your customized prescription. You'll be well on the way to feeling like your best self again, and empowered in taking back control of your health and well-being.

This part of life is a transitional journey that can take two to ten years, so get ready to check-in periodically (at least annually) for more testing and a possible new prescription. As your body changes, its need for the different hormones in varying combinations will change.

What is a compound pharmacy?

Compounding pharmacies are just that: they combine and/or alter ingredients to make a customized product for patients. These medications are compounded in response to a licensed practitioner's prescription, which has been individualized for the customer. Your bio-identicals may come in a cream, a lozenge, a patch, or pellets placed under your skin, as there are multiple ways to get the hormone replacements into your bloodstream where they do you the most good.

Fantastic Four # 4: Sleep

Sleep is one of the new darlings of the healthier living and weight loss space. With Arianna Huffington's book *The Sleep Revolution*, where she boldly claims we are in a sleep crisis (16), issues surrounding sleep have hit the mainstream.

Finally, we are talking about the importance of sleep and moving away from that insane concept that we can just keep on working and doing more, all hours of the day and night. NO! Our bodies, our minds, and our souls must have rest, downtime, the ability to recharge and restore from the myriad of thoughts, activities, and demands of our days. In fact, most of the population needs 7-8 hours of sleep every 24 hours. We need it for stress relief and body homeostasis—where all our systems are working optimally so we are ready and fresh to hit it the next day.

Sleep is measured by how many hours we sleep, how often we wake up in the middle of the sleep, and how easy or difficult it is to go to sleep and get back to sleep when disrupted. You know you need more sleep if you wake up still exhausted, with that groggy, pulling through mud feeling. So many of our choices are negatively affected if we have poor sleep. Research shows we make poorer food choices, we tend to be more sedentary and move less, we are easily irritated or overwhelmed. Chronic lack of sleep may be more harmful to women than men by producing stronger negative consequences (17). These include increased stress, increased anger and depression, increased risk for high blood pressure and obesity, and increased levels of C-Reactive Protein (C-RP) and IL-1, which are cellular mediators associated with heart disease and higher levels of blood insulin. These are all major health concerns we want to avoid. And to top it all off, sleep plays a major role in the production of hormones—those that control our mood and metabolism, organ functions, and energy levels. To beat the Hormone Groan, we need to get our sleep.

Tips for sleep hygiene

Even the name is new and cool. Sleep Hygiene. From the National Sleep Foundations website, here's the definition:

"Sleep hygiene is a variety of different practices that are necessary to have normal, quality nighttime sleep and full daytime alertness" (18).

Sleep Hygiene practices: The most important sleep hygiene practices are the ones you work to control in the environment around you. This is empowering! You can help to beat the Hormone Groan with the very things you do to get ready for bed each night. Just like the routines we engage in with very young children, doing certain things every night to get them ready for bed and sleep, we need to do for ourselves. Have a getting-ready-for-sleep routine. Below are some of the top tips all sleep professionals, blogs, and books recommend.

Melatonin: This occurs naturally in your brain and helps control your sleep /wake cycle. Levels generally peak in the evening, which help you to fall asleep. It is greatly affected and regulated by the light and dark cycles of the day and night. This is why sleeping in a dark room is important, as is getting into light first thing in the morning. It helps to regulate your melatonin levels. This also is why it is recommended to have no electronics in your face at least 30 minutes before your bed time. Melatonin levels are affected by what is coming in to your eyes, through your pupils to the retina and the light from TV, computers, phones, and tablets are detrimental to your body's natural sleep cycle. The artificial light from your devices is seen as daylight, so the brain doesn't release melatonin.

Getting ready for sleep time, the body wants those signals of relaxing, shutting down the work center, the darker or lower light, and softer sounds—all these environmental factors are important to your melatonin levels and ultimately your sleep success. Taking a melatonin supplement in the evening can also help with your body's sleep cycle. According to our favorite Web MD, it is ok to use a melatonin supplement short or long term (19). If we can get what we need from the natural environment of light vs. darkness, the melatonin would just be that—a supplement to our natural rhythms.

Reduce alcohol and heavy meals before bed: If you like cocktails or glasses of wine or beer in the evening as I do, it is helpful to your sleep cycle to stop drinking alcohol at least two to three hours before bedtime. I know how hard it is to do that, especially if you are drinking with friends and enjoying the evening. Or experimenting with some of the martini recipes in this book. Or attending conferences and meetings in different time zones, where late night meals with wine are the norm. Whatever your circumstances, drinking alcohol up until bedtime, and eating heavy meals late at night, are bad ideas if you want a good night's sleep.

Your body cannot get to rest if it is working hard to digest food or process alcohol. You may experience bloating, gas, and acid reflux instead of sleep.

Alcohol has a rebound effect, meaning it sometimes helps you get to sleep initially, because it is a depressant, but as the body metabolizes the alcohol, blood sugar levels are impacted, insulin levels are raised, and your brain wakes up (20). And not in the clear-as-a-bell, I've-had-enough-sleep either. The waking is disruptive and it is often hard to fall back asleep afterwards.

A tip I employ is, if I've had a night where alcohol is part of the fun—a celebratory dinner, a girl's night out, a we-have-to-meet-and-commiserate-after-this-extremely-stressful-work-week, I try to switch to water at least an hour before bedtime (lots of water, two or three glasses.) This helps dilute the alcohols earlier, and gives your body a break from calories needing to be digested. My preference is warm water in the evening, as it feels very soothing to the stomach.

Make your bedroom a sanctuary: It's your place to relax. Somewhere you like to be, that signals to you it is time to unwind and get ready for sleep. Choose colors, fabrics, furniture, clean space—whatever it is that speaks relaxation to you. Remember all the tips about pleasing your senses for calmness, relaxation, and mental health? Well, make your bedroom that place that pleases you. How it looks, how it smells, how it feels. There is an entire industry out there devoted to this, and it is worth some of our time and effort to create that pleasing, relaxing space.

Sleep in complete darkness: If your bedroom has light leaking in from windows, or skylights, from clocks or devices plugged in, blackout curtains may help. Wearing an eye mask is also a wonderful way to make the room instantly dark. I use them at home, when my husband wants to stay up reading and I want to sleep, when the full moon in winter reflects too much light into the room, or when I need to nap for 15 minutes in the middle of the day—pop on the mask and I get instant, complete darkness. It has become an affectionate joke between us, as he calls me "bug" and I drop off to la-la-land.

Sleep in loose fitting or no clothes: Whatever floats your boat here. Avoid wearing night clothes that twist and tangle around your legs and body as you move during the night. Whatever you can do to lessen sleep distractions is a positive. During perimenopause, many women discover for the first time in their lives how freeing it is to sleep naked. The feel of the sheets on your skin can be luxurious, and there is no distraction of clothes getting wet during the deluges of night sweats; it just rolls off the skin onto the sheets. (Keeping sheets dry is another issue, see the chapter on night sweats).

Keep your bedroom slightly cool: Even if you need to pile on the covers, cooler air in the bedroom has been proven to help with deeper, more satisfied sleeping. I love the feeling of heavy covers on my body that get me all toasty warm, while the cooler air in the room is slightly below comfortable.

Work to regulate your sleeping hours: Go to bed and get up at the same times each day/night cycle. Try this even on your days off, as the regulation helps the body be consistently ready for sleep and waking.

Turn on or see natural light first thing upon waking: This signals to the brain that it is time to wake-up. I am especially grateful for this tip when I am travelling in a different time zone. Often, I will arrive in a city the night before an event, go to bed my regular time for that time zone, and then get up at, say, 6 am. However, to my body that 6 am is 3 or 4 am, depending on what part of the country I am in. Getting up that first morning is always BRUTAL, and the first thing I do as I peel out of bed is to turn on every light in the hotel room. It is usually always still dark outside, and I need that light to signal to my jet-lagged brain, "Time to wake up!!"

Bright light therapy boxes can provide that wake-up light if you live in a part of the planet where you have to consistently get up in the dark.

Shut down: Get away from the electronic screens at least 30 minutes before bedtime. I don't even want to fight you on this! I can't make you do it, so if you want to watch TV in your bed, or check your email one-last-time before shutting off the lights, I can't stop you. But it's not just me telling you—all sleep gurus recommend this. Your body and brain need the time to unplug and it's that light issue again—the melatonin levels. And this next one goes right along with this.

No computer or TV in the bedroom: This is also hard for many people, but it has to do with unplugging your brain from the flickering lights, not to mention content you may be consuming that is keeping the brain awake and activated, your emotions flowing, when you should be shutting down that kind of stimulation to get ready for sleep (21).

When my husband got his first iPhone, he was in love! Because his phone cover was bright pink, I named her Pinkie. Pinkie went everywhere with my husband—he could not be away from her for a minute. He was smitten. He spent every free moment learning about her systems, figuring out all the cool things she could do for him. He was enamored. I wasn't too jealous of Pinkie, because there are definitely things I share with him that she can't do.

But I had a very clear sleep hygiene routine, and firmly believed that electronics had no place in the bedroom. During that first week, things were OK. But one night, when I was all cozy in my bed, and had just finished my meditation for the night—where I go through the day in my mind, assess how things went, give up any negatives to the universe, and practice gratefulness, putting my mind and soul at peace... my husband came bounding into the bedroom and launched himself across the bed, shoving Pinkie right in my face, and started jabbering on about how cool this app he had just discovered was! His enthusiasm was bubbling over; the five-year-old-boy-delight-of-just-getting-a-new-puppy was exploding from him. My zen was shattered. My peace and calm and quieting of my mind for sleep was instantly and greatly disturbed. I had a choice to make in that moment. I could get mad and let my pounding heart escape through harsh words, or I could breathe and share in this moment of joy with my husband. I did the latter (yeah, major good wife points), but determined to make myself clear the next day when I was calmer. I did just that. The next day, in a relaxed tone of voice, I referenced the night before, reiterated to my husband how important my sleep hygiene was, how much I loved him, and how accepting I had been towards his new plaything, but I had to draw the line. Pinkie was never allowed in our bed again.

He took it pretty well, and she made sure to stay out of my bedroom.

Try to get seven to nine hours of sleep a night: I know, for those of you burning the candles at both ends this seems CRAZY, but work towards it. What can you put off until another day? Honor what your body and brain are telling you about being tired and needing rest. Most of us work hard, long hours to accomplish what we need to do any given day and the inbox is never empty.

A mantra I use at the end of the day, when there are still things on the to-do list (news flash: there always will be) is: "I have done all I could do today, and it is enough." Just thinking that or saying it out loud brings me a measure of peace and calmness.

The bedroom is for sleep: Make this place a dedicated space where you can relax, restore, and get the rest you need. Your body and brain will thank you.

Here is my Sleep Hygiene Routine. Pay special attention to the envisioning I do at the end of each day. This practice lowers my stress levels and gets my mind ready for a good night's sleep. Feel free to copy the practice.

Kelli's Sleep Hygiene Routine

An hour before bedtime:
I stop all electronics at least 30 minutes before bed.

I stop drinking alcohol at least one hour before bed.

I drink a big glass of water.

I stop answering my phone.

I stop eating.

I take my nighttime supplements (progesterone and melatonin).

I wash my face and brush my teeth.

I apply a deliciously scented lotion to my skin.

I turn off all lights in my bedroom except the lamp by my bedside.

Once in bed, I breathe deeply, close my eyes, and play back my day. Anything that was unpleasant or particularly stressful, I mentally breathe out and let go of. I then think about the good parts of the day, and I make a mental list of all that I am grateful for. After that, I turn my mind to tomorrow, and imagine the day in my head, what I will do and what successes I will have, putting a positive vibe out into the universe about tomorrow.

I pick up my book, and read until ready for sleep.

The Fantastic Four—exercise, positive food choices, hormone replacement therapy, and sleep—are the foundation for reducing or alleviating almost every symptom a woman has during this transitional time of perimenopause. Wherever you are in your menopausal journey—just starting, in the midst of it all, or post—these superpower strategies will help you live your best self. If you can commit to working on these four areas, picking a couple of things you can adjust or modify, you will have the power to change your life and to escape the Hormone Hostage Zone.

Notes

Chapter 1: Brain Fog

1. 'Brain Fog' of Menopause Confirmed. (2012). *University of Rochester Medical Center Newsroom*. www.urmc.rochester.edu/news/story/3436/brain-fog-of-menopause-confirmed.aspx.

2. Barth, C., Villringer, A., & Sacher, J. (2015). Sex Hormones Affect Neurotransmitters and Shape the Adult Female Brain during Hormonal Transition Periods. *Frontiers in Neuroscience*, 9, 37. http://doi.org/10.3389/fnins.2015.00037.

3. Karlamangla, Arun S. et al. (2017). Evidence for Cognitive Aging in Midlife Women: Study of Women's Health Across the Nation. Ed. Hemachandra Reddy. *PLoS ONE*, 12, 1. http://doi.org/10.1371/journal.pone.0169008.

4. Morris, Susan York. (2017). Does Menopause Cause Memory Loss? *Healthline*. www.healthline.com/health/menopause-and-memory-loss.

5. Brizendine, L. (2006). *The Female Brain*. Broadway Books

Chapter 2: The Bitch!

1. Komaroth, Anthony L. The Gut-Brain Connection. Healthbeat. *Harvard Health Publications, Harvard Medical School*. www.health.harvard.edu/diseases-and-conditions/the-gut-brain-connection.

2. http://emerita.com/featured-products.html/

3. Powers, J. (2012) *Oh, Shift!* Powerhouse, Inc.

4. Here is just one great website I use for meditation: how-to-meditate.org/breathing-meditations

Chapter 3: Basement Blues

1. Rekkas, Paraskevi Vivien, et al. (2014). Greater monoamine oxidase A binding in perimenopausal age as measured with carbon 11–labeled harmine positron emission tomography. *JAMA Psychiatry*, 71, 8, pp. 873-879.

2. Kerr, M. (2012). Perimenopausal Depression. *Healthline*. www.healthline.com/health/depression/perimenopausal-depression

3. Romain, T. (2014). *If You Don't Take Care of Your Body, Where Else Are You Going to Live?* Porchlight Home Entertainment.

4. Pendry, L. F. & Salvatore, J. (2015). Individual and social benefits of online discussion forums. *Computers in Human Behavior*, 50, pp. 211-220.

5. *Depression & Menopause*. (2017). The North American Menopause Society. www.menopause.org/for-women/menopauseflashes/mental-health-at-menopause/depression-menopause

6. Freeman, E.W. et al. (2011). Efficacy of Escitalopram for Hot Flashes in Healthy Menopausal Women: A Randomized Controlled Trial. *JAMA*, 305, 3, pp. 267–274. doi:10.1001/jama.2010.2016

7. Find a Menopause Practitioner. (2017). *The North American Menopause Society*. www.menopause.org/for-women/find-a-menopause-practitioner.

8. Jacka, Felice N., et al. (2010). Association of Western and traditional diets with depression and anxiety in women. *American Journal of Psychiatry*, 167, 3, pp. 305-311. doi.org/10.1176/appi.ajp.2009.09060881

9. Scaccia, A. (2016). Is a Vitamin D Deficiency Causing Your Depression? *Healthline*. www.healthline.com/health/depression-and-vitamin-d.

Chapter 4: Periods Unleashed

1. Pick, M. (2013). *Is It Me or My Hormones?* Hay House, Inc.

2. Northrup, C. (2006). *The Wisdom of Menopause.* Bantam Books.

3. https://www.menopause.org/for-women/menopauseflashes/
    menopause-symptoms-and-treatments/how-do-i-know-i%27m-in-
    menopause. How Do I Know I'm In Menopause? (2017). *The North
    American Menopause Society.*

4. Mayo Clinic Staff. (2017). Perimenopause. *Mayo Clinic.* www.
    mayoclinic.org/diseases-conditions/perimenopause/diagnosis-
    treatment/diagnosis/dxc-20253805

5. Williams, V. (2017). Mayo Clinic Minute: Birth control and
    perimenopause. *Mayo Clinic.* newsnetwork.mayoclinic.org/discussion/
    mayo-clinic-minute-birth-control-and-perimenopause/

Chapter 5: The Hot Flash

1. Hot-flashes. (2017) Rvd. by Krucik, G. *Healthline.* www.healthline.
    com/symptom/hot-flashes

2. Mayo Clinic Staff. (2017). Hot Flashes. *Mayo Clinic.* www.mayoclinic.
    org/diseases-conditions/hot-flashes/symptoms-causes/dxc-20319436

3. (See Chapter 4, Entry 6)

4. Herbs and Phytoestrogens. (2015). *National Woman's Health Network.*
    www.nwhn.org/herbs-and-phytoestrogens/

5. Bailey, T.G., et al. (2016). Exercise Training Reduces the Frequency
    of Menopausal Hot Flushes By Improving Thermoregulatory Control.
    Medscape. www.medscape.com/viewarticle/ 865794_1

6. Hammar, M., et al. (1995). The Effects of Physical Activity on

Menopausal Symptoms and Metabolic Changes around Menopause. *The Journal of The North American Menopause Society,* 2, 4 pp. 201-209. journals.lww.com/menopausejournal/ Abstract/1995/02040/ The_Effects_of_Physical_Activity_on_Menopausal.4.aspx

7.   Bailey T et al (2015) Exercise training reduces the acute physiological severity of post-menopausal hot flushe. doi: 10.1113/JP271456 http://onlinelibrary.wiley.com/doi/10.1113/JP271456/full

8.   Franco, O.H. (2016). Use of Plant-Based Therapies and Menopausal Symptoms, *JAMA,* 315, 23. pp. 2554-2563. doi:10.1001/jama.2016.8012

9.   (See Chapter 2, Entry 4)

Chapter 6: Night Sweats

1.   http://www.drnorthrup.com/hot-flashes/

2.   Rabbitt, M. (2016). 3 Simple Breathing Exercises That Ease Hot Flashes. Prevention. www.prevention.com/health/breathing-exercises-to-ease-hot-flashes

3.   Boyles, S. (2012). Menopause: Smokers Have More Hot Flashes. WebMD. www.webmd.com/women/news/20120503/menopause-smokers-have-more-hot-flashes

4.   Best 5 Tips to Help You Cope with Night Sweats. (2017). 34 Menopause Symptoms. www.34-menopause-symptoms.com/night-sweats/articles/best-5-tips-to-help-you-cope-with-night-sweats.htm

5.   https://www.ncbi.nlm.nih.gov/pubmed/9694408

Chapter 7: I Want My Wine and Chips

1. McCulloch, M. (2015). Appetite Hormones. *Today's Dietitian,* 17, 70, p. 26. www.todaysdietitian.com/newarchives/070115p26.shtml

2. Wurtman, J. (2017). The Antidepressant Diet. *Psychology Today.* www.psychologytoday.com/blog/the-antidepressant-diet/201008/seroto

3. Elkaim, Y. (2014). This is Why You Have Food Cravings. *U.S. News and World Report.* health.usnews.com/health-news/blogs/eat-run/2014/03/21/this-is-why-you-have-food-cravings

4. Conger, C. (2017). How Food Cravings Work. *HowStuffWorks.* science.howstuffworks.com/innovation/edible-innovations/food-craving1.htm

5. Bouchez, C. (2017). Serotonin: 9 Questions and Answers. *WebMD.* www.webmd.com/depression/features/serotonin#3

6. Young, S. N. (2007). How to increase serotonin in the human brain without drugs. *Journal of Psychiatry & Neuroscience,* 32, 6, pp. 394-399. www.ncbi.nlm.nih.gov/pmc/articles/PMC2077351/

7. https://www.webmd.com/diet/features/water-for-weight-loss-diet#2

Chapter 8: Back Fat and Jelly Rolls

1. https://news.ohsu.edu/2003/11/07/ohsu-researchers-reveal-relationship-between-weight-gain-and-hormones

2. The Active Times. (2014). Sitting Is the New Smoking: Ways a Sedentary Lifestyle Is Killing You. *HUFFPOST.* www.huffingtonpost.com/the-active-times/sitting-is-the-new-smokin_b_5890006.html

3. Yvonne R. (2009). Weight Gain in Menopause is Preventable. *Ezinearticles.* ezinearticles.com/?Weight-Gain-in-Menopause-is-Preventable&id=3031954

4. http://www.mayoclinic.org/healthy-lifestyle/womens-health/
    in-depth/menopause-weight-gain/art-20046058?pg=2
5. https://www.psychologytoday.com/blog/real-healing/201307/the-
    menopausal-15-warding-mid-life-weight-gain
6. Marchione, M. (2015). Scientists discover how key gene makes people
    fat. *USA Today*. www.usatoday.com/story/news/ health/2015/08/ 19/
    obesity-gene/32026927/
7. Kirkpatrick, K. (2015). Avoid These Ten Foods Full of Trans Fats.
    Cleveland Clinic. health.clevelandclinic.org/2015/07/avoid-these-10-
    foods-full-of-trans-fats/
8. Joo, Eun Yeon, et al. (2012). Adverse effects of 24 hours
    of sleep deprivation on cognition and stress hormones.
    Journal of Clinical Neurology, 8, 2 pp.146-150. synapse.
    koreamed.org/search.php? where=aview&id=10.3988/
    jcn.2012.8.2.146&code=0145JCN&vmode=FULL
9. Fung, J. (2016). *The Obesity Code*. Greystone Books.
10. Zelman, K. M. (2017). Foods That Curb Hunger. *WebMD*. www.webmd.
    com/ diet/obesity/features/foods-that-curb-hunger
11. Burke, L. E. (2011). Self-Monitoring in Weight Loss: A Systematic
    Review of the Literature. *PubMed Central*. www.ncbi.nlm.nih.gov/pmc/
    articles/ PMC3268700/

Chapter 9: Mouth on Fire

1. Menopause Guidebook. (2017). *The North American Menopause
    Society*. www.menopause.org/publications/consumer-publications/-
    em-menopause-guidebook-em-8th-edition http://www.menopause.
    org/publications/clinical-care-recommendations/chapter-2-midlife-

body-changes

2. Geographic Tongue. (2015). Prpd. by Radfar, L. *The American Academy of Oral Medicine.* www.aaom.com/index.php?option=com_content&view=article&id= 131:geographic-tongue&catid=22:patient-condition-information&Itemid=120

3. https://www.ncbi.nlm.nih.gov/pmc/articles/PMC3570906/

4. http://www.mouthhealthy.org/en/az-topics/h/hormones

5. http://www.joponline.org/doi/abs/10.1902/jop.2008.080233

6. Rosania, Low, McCormick, et al. (2009). Stress, Depression, Cortisol, and Periodontal Disease. *Journal of Periodontology*, 80:2, 260-266

7. Herlofson B.B., Barkvoll, P. (1994). Sodium lauryl sulfate and recurrent aphthous ulcers. A preliminary study. *PebMed Central.* www.ncbi.nlm.nih.gov/pubmed/7825393

8. Vitamin B12 Dietary Supplement Fact Sheet. (2016). *National Institute of Health Office of Dietary Supplements.* ods.od.nih.gov/factsheets/VitaminB12-HealthProfessional/

9. Antinoro, L. (2015). Getting Enough Vitamin B12. *HEALTHbeat.* Harvard Health Publications, Harvard Medical School. www.health.harvard.edu/vitamins-and-supplements/getting-enough-vitamin-b12

Chapter 10: Let's Talk About Sex, Baby

1. Faubion, S. S. (2016). *Mayo Clinic: The Menopause Solution: A doctor's guide to relieving hot flashes, enjoying better sex, sleeping well, controlling your weight, and being happy!* Time Books, Inc. https://www.womenshealthnetwork.com/sexandfertility/menopause-sexdrive-libido.aspx

2. Northrup, C. (2006) *The Wisdom of Menopause*, pp. 276-307.

Bantam Books.

3.   Cutler, W. B. (2009). Hormones and Your Health, pp. 233-256. John Wiley & Sons, Inc.

4.   Dr. Barb. (2017). The Recipe for Sexual Health. *MiddlesexMD*. middlesexmd.com/pages/understand-the-recipe

5.   Jaecks, K. S. (2007). Got Masturbation?: A Feminist Critique of Betty Dodson's 'Sex Coaching'. *Northwest Communication Association Annual Conference.*

6.   Ibid. (2006). Women, Sex Toys and Home Parties: A Curious Revolution. *Northwest Communication Association Annual Conference.*

Fantastic Four

1.   Hammer, Matts, Brynhildsen, et al. (1995). The Effects of Physical Activity on Menopausal Symptoms and Metabolic Changes around Menopause. *Menopause*,2,4, pp. 201-209

2.   Food Allergies: What You Need to Know. (2017). U.S. *Food and Drug Administration*. www.fda.gov/food/resourcesforyou/ consumers/ ucm079311.htm

3.   Healthy Aging. (2017). *John Hopkins Medicine*. www.hopkinsmedicine. org/health/healthy_aging/healthy_body/the-brain-gut-connection

4.   Sonnenburg, E. & Sonnenburg, J. (2015). Gut Feelings–the "Second Brain" in Our Gastrointestinal Systems [Excerpt]. *Scientific American*. www.scientificamerican.com/ article/gut-feelings-the-second-brain-in-our-gastrointestinal-systems-excerpt/

5.   Evrensel A. & Ceylan M.E. (2015). The Gut-Brain Axis: The Missing Link in Depression. *Clinical Psychopharmacology and Neuroscience*, 13, 3, pp. 239-244. doi:10.9758/cpn.2015.13.3.239

6. Hemarajata, P. & Versalovic, J. (2013). Effects of probiotics on gut microbiota: mechanisms of intestinal immunomodulation and neuromodulation. *Therapeutic Advances in Gastroenterology*, 6, 1, pp. 39-51. doi:10.1177/1756283X12459294

7. Whole Grains and Fiber. (2017). *American Heart Association*. www.heart.org/HEARTORG/ HealthyLiving/HealthyEating/ HealthyDietGoals/Whole-Grains-and-Fiber_UCM_303249_ Article. jsp#.WYOhFK2ZOu4

8. The Facts on Omega-3 Fatty Acids. (2017). *WebMD*. www.webmd.com/ healthy-aging/omega-3-fatty-acids-fact-sheet

9. Rao T.S.S. et al. (2008) Understanding nutrition, depression and mental illnesses. *Indian Journal of Psychiatry*, 50, 2, pp. 77-82. doi:10.4103/0019-5545.42391

10. (see Chapter 9, Entry 8)

11. (see Chapter 9, Entry 9)

12. (see Chapter 3, Entry 9)

13. Vitamin D Dietary Supplement Fact Sheet. (2016). *National Institute of Health Office of Dietary Supplements*. ods.od.nih.gov/factsheets/ VitaminD-HealthProfessional/

14. Ritter, S. (2005). Premarin. *Chemical & Engineering News*. pubs.acs. org/cen/coverstory/83/8325/8325premarin.html

15. Brower V. A. (2003). A second chance for hormone replacement therapy? *EMBO Reports*, 4, 12, pp. 1112-1115. doi:10.1038/ sj.embor.7400043

16. Huffington, A. (2016). *The Sleep Revolution*. Christabella, LLC.

17. Soong, J. (2010). How Sleep Loss Affects Women More Than Men. *WebMD*. www.webmd.com/women/features/how-sleep-loss-affects-women-more-than-men#

18. Sleep Hygiene. (2017). *National Sleep Foundation*. sleepfoundation.
org/sleep-topics/sleep-hygiene

19. Melatonin – Overview. (2017). *WebMD*. www.webmd.com/ sleep-
disorders/tc/melatonin-overview

20. MedicineNet. (2007). Q. How does alcohol affect blood sugar?
WebMDanswers. answers.webmd.com/answers/1166930/how-does-
alcohol-affect-blood-sugar

21. Healthy Sleep Tips. (2017). *National Sleep Foundation*.
sleepfoundation.org/sleep-tools-tips/healthy-sleep-tips/page/0/1

Kelli welcomes your stories, comments, and questions about your menopause journey. Please connect with her at:
Kellijaecks.com

LINKEDIN
Kelli Swanson Jaecks, MA, RDH
www.linkedin.com/in/kellijaecks

FACEBOOK
Kelli Jaecks Verbal Impact
@kellijaecks

INSTAGRAM
@kellijaecksverbalimpact

Let's Soirée!

Kelli Jaecks may soon be coming to your town!

What is a Martinis & Menopause Soirée?

A soirée is a social event held in private homes or at local area businesses in cities across the United States that combines a cocktail-party atmosphere with valuable, practical information. These fun, educational, women-celebrated events create a setting that encourages open dialogue on women's health and wellness issues; focusing on perimenopause, menopause, and post-menopause.

If you are interested in throwing a soirée at your home or business and would like Kelli to speak or attend, please email your request to hello@kellijaecks.com

Additional Resources

for your next book club or event can be found at:
martinisandmenopause.com
or
kellijaecks.com

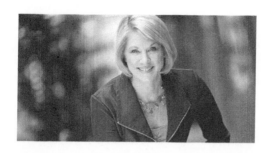

About the Author

Kelli Jaecks is a prolific speaker, blogger, and lover of life! *Martinis & Menopause* was inspired by her own journey through menopause and her passion for helping women feel better and live better. When not speaking or writing, Kelli enjoys performing in live theater and traveling to cool venues for scuba diving. She lives in Oregon with her husband. To learn more, visit kellijaecks.com.

@kellijaecks
@kellijaecksverbalimpact